MW01469829

What Remains: Breast Cancer, Mastectomy and Getting on With Life

Beth R. Minear

authorHOUSE®

AuthorHouse™
1663 Liberty Drive
Bloomington, IN 47403
www.authorhouse.com
Phone: 1 (800) 839-8640

© 2015 Beth R. Minear. All rights reserved.

No part of this book may be reproduced, stored in a retrieval system, or transmitted by any means without the written permission of the author.

Published by AuthorHouse   06/19/2015

ISBN: 978-1-5049-1803-9 (sc)
ISBN: 978-1-5049-1804-6 (hc)
ISBN: 978-1-5049-1802-2 (e)

Library of Congress Control Number: 2015909550

Print information available on the last page.

Any people depicted in stock imagery provided by Thinkstock are models, and such images are being used for illustrative purposes only.
Certain stock imagery © Thinkstock.

This book is printed on acid-free paper.

Because of the dynamic nature of the Internet, any web addresses or links contained in this book may have changed since publication and may no longer be valid. The views expressed in this work are solely those of the author and do not necessarily reflect the views of the publisher, and the publisher hereby disclaims any responsibility for them.

FORWORD AND ACKNOWLEDGEMENTS

When you are handed a diagnosis like Breast Cancer, nothing is ever the same again. Pick your cliché . . . "rug pulled out from under you"; "blind-sided"; "knocked for a loop" . . . combine them all and multiply times infinity and you may come close to the utter disbelief that follows. For me, my diagnosis came after years of annual mammograms and no family history. In the days that followed, from the date I "knew" even until the present, I've struggled to keep my equilibrium, making the tough choices when I needed to and asking for help when I needed that, too . . . and surrendering to God throughout.

This book is intended to give information to women (and men) who are going through breast cancer. It gives voice to the fears that dare not be spoken out loud and to the joy that can be yours again – a different joy, but true joy nonetheless. My story was written to share the innocence lost and wisdom gained along the way, and to give hope to those who may have misplaced theirs. If your reading this, please know that your hope isn't lost. It's still there – you sometimes need help in finding it.

I've been fortunate throughout my "journey", if that's what it is. I've been blessed with an understanding family, great friends, amazing healthcare and strangers who felt like family in the Twitterverse. One of my prayerful friends on Twitter is Rebekah Hallberg. In fall 2011, we bonded over our children who have special needs and our faith and have maintained our connection ever since. After I shared my diagnosis, although we'd never met in person, Rebekah sent some comfort items to me in the mail.

One of them was a small journal. From indecipherable scratchings made through pain medication and a heavily bandaged body, to irreverent, inappropriate thoughts jotted in the middle of the night, this book took shape. Thank you, Rebekah, for planting the seed.

I also want to thank some of the best friends that anyone could ever ask for. I've never had a gaggle of girlfriends or moved around in large circles. I admire people who have that, but it's not me. From the moment of my diagnosis, I've had near-strangers reach out to me with soft pillows to soothe radiation burns, a prayer blanket passed along from a Survivor in another state (and which I've since passed along), scarves coming in from everywhere to cover my bald head and prayers coming to me in warm waves from all over the world. "Thank you" to you all – I could feel them and they sustained me during times of despair.

I'm grateful for my family - for my mother, Deanna Lewis, and my sister, Tana Stanley, for my late father, Michael Lewis, and his wife, Mino. They knew what to say and when to be there. The love, prayers, cards, texts and rooting from the sidelines during my battle. No one has had better cheerleaders under any circumstance. My sweet dad, as he was losing his own battle with cancer, reached out to hold my hand when we were sitting on his couch three months after his brain surgery and one month after my mastectomy. "You're going to survive your cancer," he said. Thank you, Poppy, for being selfless and giving your hope to me. For my in-laws, Bill and Eleanor Minear, and the loving Minear family that I married into, I am grateful for your love.

I've also had friends who committed themselves to my care and that of my family. None more so than Deanna Taylor-Pitman and her family – "Nurse Helga" as you read. Of all of my friends, Deanna is the most like me in temperament and resourcefulness. I needed tough, when I was too weak to think, and someone to take over when chemotherapy scrambled my brains. Deanna kept me as "me" when I was in danger of losing myself and fed myself back to me as I regained my strength. I don't know what I did to deserve her and her family, but I thank God for all of them every day.

I want to thank my editor Kathryn E. Brown, Managing Member of The Write Word, LLC. Katy and I met through professional networking almost two decades ago and have been friends ever since. It was humbling to submit my work to her for critique and review, when I had admired her skills for so long as a professional editor and writer (and an author herself). There was no one else who I could trust with my story. Katy was with me throughout diagnosis and treatment, keeping in touch and keeping me in touch with the rest of our community. I knew she could apply her considerable talent to editing my manuscript without losing my voice in it. My faith was well-placed.

I also want to mention the amazing medical care that I've received along the way. It isn't lost on me how fortunate I am to live in the United States, with the best healthcare in the world. Even here in Charleston, West Virginia, I had state-of-the-art treatments, including the latest drug trials and, other than for the initial surgery, slept in my own bed every night. From the moment I found the lump to today, so many doctors, nurses, assistants, schedulers, office staff, volunteers, etc., in so many offices have all worked together as one powerful force against cancer. For me and for so many others that it hurts to think about, but I am blessed to have you on my team.

I'd like to thank two doctors in particular. One is my surgeon, Dr. Todd Witsberger, who is gifted and patient. From the moment of my first biopsy, through tests, surgery and follow ups, I truly believe that it hurt him almost as much as it did me. For anyone who lives anywhere near Charleston, when asked who my surgeon was, his name always brings a smile and a nod acknowledging my good fortune.

The other is Dr. Steven Jubelirer. To be technically correct, he is my Oncologist, but who he has been to me defies definition. Dr. Jubelirer has been the center of my treatment universe for almost three years, as of this writing. He works in tandem with the National Cancer Institute in providing the world's best cancer treatments for his patients. Quiet and brilliant, Dr. Jubelirer gives all of himself to his patients, lending quiet humor, preserving what remains of tattered modesty and a boost to the patient's battered psyche. I came through the darkness and into the light on the other side by God's grace, but was carried there in the arms of this great doctor and the support of his team at the David Lee Cancer Center. I hope to prove myself worthy of the care you have given to me.

I also want to give special thanks for Karen Pitrolo with the Center for Cancer Research – CAMC Institute. Karen is proof that angels walk among us. From the moment I met her, my heart recognized a kindred in hers and I trusted her with my life. Karen coordinated tests and examinations with lightning speed to get me approved for and randomized into a clinical trial that we chose and in time to start my first chemotheraphy treatment right on schedule. More importantly, she made me e-mail her every single day from September 5, 2012, to January 9, 2013, keeping up with the minutiae of bodily indignities that accompany such treatments. Her daily responses were thoughtful, heartfelt and spiritual as she cared for me through hell and back. As strange as this sounds, I am grateful to cancer for bringing Karen into my life.

To my boys. Billy, my stepson, who I couldn't love any more than I do. You have grown into such a loving and thoughtful man. I appreciate the love and support that you have given to me, but, more so, I appreciate the quiet strength that you gave to your dad during my treatments. I am so proud of you. To David, my sweet son, you are the light of my life. The reason I was born was to be your mother. Every decision made during this nightmare was made knowing that I had to be around to see you grow up. You are such a special kid, and your dad and I can't wait to see you change the world.

Finally, to my strong, sensitive husband, Bill . . . my Love. I have no words to convey what you are to me. From the moment we met, I knew that you were the only man that I could forever be with. I felt guilty over my diagnosis and worried about what my treatment was taking out of you. You never complained, never wavered in your love for me. It takes a special man to look at his post-mastectomy, gray-skinned, greasy-haired wife like she's the most beautiful woman in the world. You did that for me – for us. It's hard to imagine loving you more, but I still do – every day.

To God – all the glory to You, and praise lifted up in Your name for my life. Please be with those who are scared and suffering. Give them the strength to sustain them through the worst of their earthly trials, and let them know that peace and comfort is theirs if they will ask You for it. Amen.

June 27, 2013

Running around today, getting ready for vacation. Long-awaited and well-deserved. Going through the list of "must do"s that every mother creates before going on vacation. (Yes, I know Daddies go on vacation in many households as well, but their list is two entries long; 1) cellphone; and 2) what they're taking for themselves. Moms have the rest of it. Laundry finished . . . check. My clothes and David's clothes packed . . . check. Pick up prescriptions . . . check. Mail stopped and groceries for the trip bought . . . check and check. Oil changed, tires rotated, gas in the minivan . . . check, check, check.

All of the personal duties are in addition to my mostly 60-hour work weeks as in-house counsel for a Fortune 500 energy company. The day before, I had been in Cleveland, working though a particularly tough settlement with multiple parties in litigation with my company. The rest of the week had been in hyper-mode of 12-hour days, trying to get enough off of my plate so I wouldn't feel guilty about leaving work for a week. I don't know why I worry so much. They can survive without me and some of my colleagues take off at the drop of a hat and let everything crumble (or wait) until they get back. I've been doing better during the past year, as my priorities have definitely rearranged, but I still don't want to leave my clients and co-workers holding a bag that I should have tied off and disposed of before I left.

David ("the Buddy") and I returned from his viola lesson, a summer addition to our busy schedule. He had played the cello during his fourth grade year, but had started pining for the viola half-way through the term. We had him finish the year on cello, but picked up summer viola lessons in the hope that he could learn enough with his awesome viola instructor to be able to rejoin his classmates in the Strings for the fifth grade. After viola, the Buddy and I ran over to visit my Dad and his wife, Mino, which he loves to do, before heading for home and resuming vacation prep.

Cleaning out the minivan's cargo area proved to be a fairly quick chore – most of the "necessities" in there, such as lawn chairs, umbrellas and toys, were going with us anyway. I finished tossing the last of the water bags and drink cups, picked up the mail from the mailbox and was absent-mindedly shuffling through the bills, magazines and advertisements – and a small, innocuous-looking postcard stopped me in my tracks, halfway up the driveway. Knowing how distressed the Buddy gets when I cry, I held back the tears while that awful and now all-too-familiar ball of lead settled in my stomach. The handwriting on this postcard addressed to me was my own – the reminder for my annual mammogram. The staff at the mammography clinic have you fill out the card to yourself when you update your medical records each year.

I lost my breasts last year.
I wouldn't need a mammogram this year.
What a year it has been . . .

June 29, 2012

"Man, that wind is really blowing!" I thought. It was around dinner-time and we were getting settled for a hot weekend. The sky over Charleston had looked so strange during the past hour, like nothing I had ever seen before. It doesn't matter that we don't live in Tornado Alley, or even that West Virginia doesn't get that many tornados, or even strong ones when it does. When the wind blows the way it's blowing, I always take the Buddy and head to the basement. Bill, my husband and David's daddy, is more fascinated, than fearful. He grabs the cellphone and starts taking videos in front of the glass storm door, commenting on the decades-old Hemlocks and Oak trees, bending and whipping around. "You should really see this!" he yells, mesmerized by the storm. "I'll watch the video," I think, and watch the Buddy play with his "WALL-E" action-figures.

I'm dreading tomorrow. It's been so hot - in the high 80s, 90s and even low 100s for more than a week, this first full week of Summer 2012. Tomorrow is the last day of Corporate Cup, Charleston area YMCA's annual corporate "Olympics". It always ends with a full day of track and field at University of Charleston football stadium (previously called "Laidley Field") and we, middle-aged, long beyond glory days warriors converge on the field to compete against our peers in an obstacle course, sprints, relays, distance runs, field event, etc.. As well as I know my own name, I know that it'll be broiling on the astro-turf tomorrow, that I'll be sore for a week afterward and that I'll swear to be in better shape for next year's Cup.

"Well," I mused, as the weather raged outside, "at least this year I have better running shoes and a couple of new bras." As a 38DD, well-fitting bras that both support and strap down "the girls" have been a necessity since the DDs introduced themselves to my body at age 17. I was a 32DD then, but then, as the saying goes "my drinking-glass figure used to be an hour-glass." In talking with an equally-endowed friend at work, she had suggested that I wear two sport bras or on sport bra over my regular underwire for additional support and control. I had taken her just that a couple of days before, wrestling my mammoth (and increasingly low-hanging) breasts into the cups of both bras, one bra over the other, while squeezed into the tiny, tiny fitting rooms in the middle of Dick's.

"**BOOM . . . BOOM!**" "What was THAT?!" I thought. I had never heard anything quite like it. It sounded like the air shredded into pieces. I immediately thought of the Stephen King novella "The Langoliers" and, absurdly, my mind went to how awful the movie was compared to the book. The luxury of ruminating was short-lived as the electricity went out in the house.

"The neighborhood is dark," Bill called down, as if reading my mind. "Crap," I thought, "I hope it comes back on soon." As with most Fridays, I had stocked our refrigerator for the weekend to get it out of the way, so I was already planning how to manage the next few hours of keeping the Buddy (and Bill) out of the fridge and freezer until the power came back on.

"Thank God my iPhone and work phone are charged," I thought, knowing we'd be able to call and text and keep the Buddy entertained until the power came back on. As the wind died down, we went upstairs and found my husband at the kitchen table, checking his phone messages. Bill is the Deputy Director for Critical Infrastructure with the WV Fusion Center, having retired as the Police Chief in Williamstown, West Virginia, a few months before the Buddy was born. He's not on regular patrol anymore, but when there are potential threats to the state's critical infrastructure, man-made or like the storm, I know I may see him very little during the coming days.

I went around the house, pulling the curtains closed, trying to keep in as much of our air conditioning as possible, in case the electricity didn't come on before we went to bed. It had been more than 100 today, so opening the windows in the hopes of cooler air was not possible. None of us Minears can sleep when we're too hot, so there was the potential for a long night, although in the 12 years I had lived on Fort Hill (so named for the Civil War fort at the top where both Presidents Hayes and McKinley had served), we rarely lost power. When we did, the power company had it restored within a few hours, 12 tops during a winter storm when David was little and Bill out of town.

I called Dad and Mino to check on them. "Yep" their power was out, too. I was a little concerned for them. Dad had just had a malignant brain tumor removed on June 1, 2012, and was slowly regaining strength, stamina and his appetite. While being without air conditioning was annoying for us, it could prove much more concerning for him.

* *

During the next few days, we found that Charleston, heck, West Virginia and the surrounding states had been hit with a *fairly-rare weather phenomenon called a "Derecho", a 80 plus mile-per-hour, straight-line storm of hot air. It took out power to approximately 80 percent of the state and with it, the ability to pump gasoline, cool homes and businesses, charge cellphones and find stores open with groceries and ice. Bill was working for the first three days non-stop. Hospital generators in parts of the state were running out of gasoline and he was finding that most of the gasoline tanker refueling stations, like the one at the front of Fort Hill, were unable to tap their reserves for the first day since their power was out, too. Bill was utilizing state radio traffic to direct the tankers that needed to get fuel to the hospitals to refueling stations in other states. He was also trying to find staging areas and shelter for the thousands of out-of-state electrical workers who were coming to help us. Unlike many storms, where our neighboring states help us and vice versa, the Derecho was so wide-spread, that there were crews from half the country away, coming to our aid. Those power truck convoys were a beauty to behold.*

On the homefront, we had taken the fruit, yoghurt, milk, lunchmeat to Dad's the next day to get some value before giving the refrigerator contents up to lost. We had roughed it sleeping in the "cool" 80-degree basement, and then, blessedly, while Bill scoured the city looking for an open gas station at 5:30 a.m., I had managed to book Dad and Mino and Bill, David and me into two rooms at Embassy Suites for a few days and had stocked the tiny fridges in the rooms with provisions to make it more comfortable and less expensive than eating out. Dad was doing fine, the Buddy was entertaining him in the lobby, which had become a city-wide block-party. More natives were at the hotel than out-of-towners post-Derecho, and Dad was holding court with some folks who were happy to see him out post-surgery. Mino and I were taking turns, checking houses for electricity and running family errands. Their power came on Tuesday, July 3, so they quickly packed up and moved back home, vacating the room for other Derecho-refugees who kept pouring in when other locals returned home.

Our power didn't come back on for a few more days . . . which might have saved my life. The Derecho might have saved my life.

Mammograms

I had been going for an annual mammogram since my early 30s. No family history of breast cancer on either side for as long as anyone could peg. Colon cancer, "yes" – multiple family members on my mother's side. Ovarian cancer, "yes" – my paternal grandmother died of it in the early 80s. Dad's brain tumor, metastasized from non-smoker's lung cancer three years prior, was not hereditary. No one had had breast cancer.

I went annually because my insurance had always paid for it. Just like colonoscopies every ten years (I've done that, too), if there is a routine, preventative screening that my insurance pays for, I'm going to have it. For 13 years, my mammograms have been non-issues . . . if slamming your breasts in car doors can be considered non-issues. The staff are fantastic at making them as smooth and easy as possible.

In 2011, my mammogram had been routine. My 2012 mammogram had been scheduled for early May, but I had been travelling for work and had to reschedule the appointment. I wasn't concerned in doing so. At only 44, and no family history, mammograms were party of my "routine" checkups each year, and nothing more. Nothing more than showing up, updating my medical history, slamming my breasts in the car door . . . and addressing the reminder card to myself for the next year's exam.

July 4, 2012

Staying at the Embassy was originally an adventure for the Buddy. He loves hotels, having travelled with his daddy and me for work whenever we were able to make it a family gig. We made sure to bring his current favorites of clothes, snacks, toys and movie and he made an immediate nest in a corner of the suite, arranging things to his liking. Dad and Mino's power had come back on the day prior, so I could focus on keeping the Buddy and me afloat while Bill still worked on helping private and public infrastructure entities get back on line. Who contemplated a potential water shortage when there was plenty of water? Without electricity for water treatment, pumping, etc., folks can be out of water even when there is plenty.

Thank God, too, for the Fourth of July, this year. And not just in the patriotic, "Hell yeah, I'm proud to be an American," sense this year. During the Derecho power outage, while taking care of my family, helping Mino take care of Dad, keeping Bill on his feet from exhaustion and running home to check the neighborhood cat, Norman, the house and empty the fridge and freezer of all that food, I had still been working for the gas company, both from the office (David in tow) and the hotel. A good deal of my job entails helping internal clients with their operations and maintenance projects and with capital growth projects, the bulk of which projects are advanced in the summer. Derecho or not, the projects were moving forward. The Fourth of July gave me a one-day buffer to focus on us – on the Buddy.

We had been in and out of bathing suits all summer, at various pools, at the beach and, now, at the Embassy pool. We'd rinse *out wet suits and shuffle them with dry ones at home on our many daily checks of the house, so we were packing and unpacking the pool bag all day this Fourth. Slipping into the bathroom in our hotel room, I shrugged my way out of the bathing suit top and caught a glimpse of myself in the mirror.*

"What is THAT?!" I stared in horror. At the 3:00 position on my right breast was a dimple . . . a pull of flesh that I hadn't noticed before. Not in the tiny, tiny dressing room mirror at Dick's that week-feels-like-a-century ago, not at the beach, not once. I reached down and touched it, not knowing what to expect. Under my fingers, was a small finch-egg sized lump. Hard and unyielding, I looked in the mirror, bile rising to the back of my throat. "OmyGod, omyGod, omyGod" . . . mind racing, I racked my thoughts for any time during the past few days that I could have bumped and injured my breast. Hauling luggage, toys, books, computer in and out of the house, the hotel, work . . .? Cleaning out the refrigerator and freezer, hauling the four massive garbage bags to the dumpster that the City of Charleston blessedly installed in our neighborhood to help clean-up? Climbing in and out of the pool?

I knew it wasn't an injury – I knew it. No matter how suddenly it manifested, no matter that it wasn't there on the 2011 mammogram, I knew that the lump was a lump – it didn't belong there and wasn't going away on its own. Prayers formed in my head and silently murmured through my lips, "please don't let it be cancer, please let it be benign." But, I knew. I KNEW, as surely as I have ever known anything.

I dressed and came out of the bathroom, the Buddy lost in make-believe. I sat down and flipped on the television, watching nothing. When Bill came in, we went over to Dad and Mino's to celebrate the Fourth, bringing dinner to them so Mino would have one less thing to worry about. I said nothing. Nothing. To any of them. I can't remember a word of conversation that evening.

Back at the Embassy, we settled in and heard the tell-tale signs of fireworks from outside. Although our room was on a back corner, right across from our window, reflected in the glass of the office building across the street, was a perfect view of the fireworks for the Fourth. I snuggled behind the Buddy as he laughed and said "Wow" – sniffing the back of his blonde head and wondering if I would be there to see them with him next year.

"Calm down," I told myself. "You don't even have a diagnosis . . . don't even know that it is cancer and you are already going THERE." The fireworks heralded the beginning of the "new Beth" – the "changed Beth" – the "I had cancer, Beth - the demarcation of "before and after". I still said nothing to Bill, wanting him to sleep well, maybe the last time for a long time. I haven't slept well since that day.

July 5, 2012

The Embassy is right across the street from the imaging center where I've always gotten my annual mammogram. Bill took the Buddy with him the next morning to check on the house. I intended to go to work, but planned to walk into the mammography across the street first. I left deodorant off the morning's preparations and, when the boys left the hotel, I walked across the street and signed in. I had cancelled the scheduled appointment from six weeks ago, as I had been travelling for work, so I was (and have been since) chastising myself for missing the annual check-up.

Walking up to the second floor, taking the clipboard and filling out my medical chart update for the past year, I marvel at how lucky I had been in the health department to date. At 44 years old, other than a transient ischemic attacks or "mini- stroke" at 29 years old, during law school (birth control side effect), there was nothing remarkable about me – at all. I still had twenty pounds I wanted to loose, but, otherwise, great condition. Finalizing the update, I self-addressed my reminder post-card for next year. Even with my nerves and fears about the lump I found the day before, the irony of filling out the card was lost on my.

Walk-ins are treated well at the digital imagery center I go to. None of the stony glares, the one-word answers and clipped tones you get at many doctors' office the few times I'd squeezed the Buddy or me in for a "sick visit." Mammography caregivers really want to screen you, now, today, no appointment necessary.

Aside from the Derecho chatter, and comparisons of "is your power back on yet?" "No" or "yes, mine came on Tuesday," there was nothing different about this visit than my other dozen or so before. Not apparently for them, but it was brutal for me. They couldn't see the lump, not only dimpling and pulling at my skin, but pulling at my heart, as I was checked in and prepped for the mammogram. The same wonderful mammographer who has done my mammograms for years was there, tiny and in charge of me and the rest of her patients. We went through some catching up about family and what-not . . . why was I suddenly shy to tell her what I saw, what I found, what I feared? This was why I walked-in instead of rescheduling my missed appointment.'

"I have a lump," I blurted out. "Maybe a bumped my breast recently, injured it, or something. Maybe I have Mastitis or an infection or something." I was rambling, fearful, hopeful, prayerful that this wasn't what I thought it was. Something passed briefly through the eyes of this wonderful person who I had gone to and who had mashed, molded and tugged by 38DDs onto those plates for all these years. Was it sadness for me? Fear? Prayer? Then it was gone and with her typical efficiency, I was whisked into the screening room where films and films were taken, both of the left breast and the offending breast, as she reminded me that we didn't know anything yet and needed to wait until the radiologist read the films. She taped metal dots over the lump and took closer, tighter, squeezier photos of the area – "crush it out of there" I thought, knowing that was impossible.

Looking over my shoulder at the screen, I saw the images flash of what was being taken, of what would be electronically sent to the radiologist to read. Unmistakably, even to my untrained eye, I saw an egg-like shape, shown in neon-green, dotted relief. I had never seen that on prior mammograms and nothing remotely similar was taken from the left breast.

"Which doctors would you like to have the results, Beth?" she asked. "Definitely Dr. Gyne, my OB-GYN" I answered, "and "Dr. Joy, my family doctor, please. I have my annual gynecological exam tomorrow morning, with Dr. Gyne and will tell him to look for the results in the next few days." My long-time mammographer looked at me fiercely, kindly, and said "I can't promise, but I'm going to try to get the results to Dr. Gyne by your morning appointment." I blinked back tears, horrified at the possible implication, grateful for her compassion and, strangely, embarrassed to be in this situation. Embarrassed? Yes, but touched and grateful more so. She hugged me tightly and sent me out the door.

Later that afternoon, during one of our frequent checks, we found that our power had come back on. Embassy let us do a late check-out without charging us for another day, so we turned the air conditioner back on in the house (we had turned everything off to protect the breaker box in the event of power surges) and started dragging our accumulation of stuff from the hotel back home. Despite the hand-washing I had done during the past seven days, we still had a mound of clothing that needed to be washed, an empty refrigerator, and a house that started to smell unlived-in in a remarkably short amount of time.

The Buddy went room to room, depositing his things back in (close to) their rightful places and I was alone, with Bill, in the kitchen. As I mopped the kitchen floor, both to freshen the room and to pick up the little bit of leakage from the defrosted refrigerator, I told my sweet husband about the lump I had found *the day before, my trip that day to get a mammogram and what I feared. "I found a lump in my right breast . . ." I said haltingly. I couldn't find the words. I wanted to spare him my horror. "I had a mammogram this morning and saw a lump on that, too. They are going to try to get preliminary results by the time of my Dr. Gyne appointment tomorrow . . ." I couldn't finish.*

My husband is a former paramedic and former firefighter in addition to being a retired police chief. "Robby Rescue" as I call him. I could tell by the look on his face that he wanted to save me from my fears and from whatever had invaded me. I stood up, silent tears running down my cheeks and let Bill wrap me in that wonderful hug that he has. "We'll figure it out," he said, hugging and hugging. The Buddy walked in and, as usual, gleefully proclaimed "group hug!" as he worked his way between his daddy and me. Bill and I hugged and hugged our little family, with the Buddy oblivious to the import in those family arms.

July 6, 2012

The next morning, after another awful, fitful night of sleep, I headed to Dr. Gyne's office for my annual gynecological exam. It was Friday, and Fridays at Dr. Gynes are usually not as busy as the rest of the week. Bill and I love Dr. Gyne. My sweet husband went to the majority of obstetrical appointments with me when I was pregnant with David. Dr. Gyne is amazing, smart and kind, but he is also a former Marine who had gone to medical school after the military. He and Bill are close in age and really hit it off due to their similar backgrounds and humor.

During this appointment, I went through our normal routine of teasing the good doctor during my examination and he gave back as good as he got. "I think you left your watch in there last year, Doctor – would you look for it?" "Well, did you keep winding it for me, Beth?" Funny, easy banter after more than a decade of talking to me through my vagina and delivering my amazing son. Again, I found myself shy about telling him about the lump I found and my mammogram during the past two days.

"Did you get any results for me yesterday or this morning?" I asked. "I know it's a long-shot to get them this soon, but I found a lump on my right breast on the Fourth and had a mammogram yesterday. They were going to try to get the results to you today, but, I know it takes a few." Dr. Gyne asked his attending nurse to check to see if the results were in while he pulled the gown off of my left shoulder first. With a serious, but calm demeanor, he did his normal breast exam on the left side, checking the entire circumference and the nodes in my armpit. He replaced my left arm into my left sleeve and pulled the gown off of my right

shoulder. "Don't tell me where," he said, "let me see if I can find what you're talking about." I looked at him and said, in the same joking tone I have for him, but not-really joking, "if you can't find this lump, I need a new doctor. You can't miss it." He looked down at the dimple, at the lump, palpated it a few times and replaced the gown on the right side.

By that time, the nurse had come back in with the mammogram report. Dr. Gyne read the confusing results out loud – results that really weren't resolving anything. He said that some of the key words he looks for like "lobular" weren't in there. He said it may be nothing, as it came up so fast, as many breast cancers were slow-growing. "To be on the safe side," he said, "let's get you scheduled for a biopsy. Do you have a family surgeon? I can recommend one if you don't." I told him that we see Dr. Healer and I wanted him to do the biopsy, if he could. Dr. Gyne nodded, "I like Todd", he said, "we'll get it set up."

I left with an appointment for a biopsy for the following Thursday, July 12.

David

David's story starts normally enough. Mommy and Daddy meet at a conference in a remote part of our rural state, fall in love (truly at first sight), get married and have a baby all in less than two years. David was a big baby, 9 pounds, 5 ounces, 21 1/2 inches long with a perfectly round head. He was frank breech while I was carrying him, so I had a C-section, but he was and remains the most beautiful kid I've ever seen. Blond hair, beautiful, light blue eyes, tall, strong and with his Daddy's deep, deep dimples. David also has Asperger's which, until 2012 and the new version of the Diagnostic Statistical Manual, had a distinct diagnosis on the Autism Spectrum.

David's early months and years were largely unremarkable . . . he hit his physical milestones, laughed and played, had three words by his 1st year, spoke in two-word sentences clearly by age two, and gave little indication of anything amiss. I say "little" indication as there were some early signs of "fascinations" that are very much with him today. David loved to pull off a single sock and wave and flap it endlessly, mesmerized by the movement. For years, I would pull out a box or basket and find a single sock. He loved (and loves) ceiling fans, pinwheels, windfarms, etc. - anything with that motions. He hated (and hates) the ice crusher, vacuum, leaf blower, fire alarm, etc. - anything with overwhelming sound.

Like many children with Asperger's, David never lost the ability to speak, which so often accompanies other diagnoses on the Autism Spectrum. He has always spoken very clearly, with great word inflection and prolific vocabulary (his favorite word at age 4 was "cacophony"), and no echolalia. It was the little things like his technical, all-consuming "fascinations" and his intense aversion to some stimuli, that lead his Daddy and me to seek a diagnosis around age two and a half. The hits and misses of getting that diagnosis is another topic for another book.

Other than his preferences, the remarkable aspect of David was and remains his intellect. We listened to classical music through the "Baby Einstein" series throughout his early years. Even though abandoned six or seven years ago as he moved to more sophisticated toys, David can still hear a piece of classical music on a commercial or show and, if he's heard it before, he can tell you the composer. David knew the planets on sight and in order before the age of three. He knew them so well, that he told a worker at a museum exhibit that "Neptune not look right" - and he was correct. The depiction of Neptune for that exhibit "not look right." We were popular that day. He also loves to combine common household items, organizing into a three-D collage of something else. And David has always drawn on his white board (the best gift we ever gave him from age three to now) and began doing so in three-D shortly before age four. He drew cubes and cones and had his subject matters either partially in or walking out of his picture. Sometimes you see a foot or fingers under a line where someone is under a blanket or peeking around a corner.

From an early age, David also displayed many of the remarkable traits he continues to show. Unlike some children on the Spectrum, David is amazingly affectionate. Caregivers in different classes would report that, if you sit cross-legged on the floor, David will start backing into you to sit in the hollow of your legs. He loved and loves to be hugged. David also is extremely sensitive to distress in others (inordinate stress will cause a meltdown in him from sensory overload) and would often be seen comforting other children in the class. He also has been able to read from around age two and a half - yes we read to him almost every night, but didn't teach him. This is a great gift, but proved challenging when coupled with the nap-dropping at daycare around age two. During naptime, the caregivers had to strategically place David away from other children and away from the decorated classroom boards or he would read everything on the board, calendars and walls out loud and no one would get any sleep.

"Aspies" thrive with organization, predictability, highly technical areas so are likely to be Architects or Engineers, Inventors or work with Computers. Silicon Valley is full of them - finally, these gifted, but socially-challenged souls are real players because technology caught up with their genius AND social skills are less important. Folks with Asperger's are usually great at inventions or scientific discoveries since their brains are wired to see patterns where others miss the nuances. Currently, David wants to study Robotics, but he is also amazing at computer design and graphics. He will likely have a highly technical job, but will likely always be a little behind the curve socially. The thing is . . . social skills, to a large degree, can be taught. We practice, and he gets better and better. We know it's a marathon and not a sprint, but we have the stamina to go the distance with our son. We have been blessed with some amazing families whose children are David's age and who just accept him for him and include him. David is just "David" and there isn't any big deal about it. The older he gets, the less effort it takes for him to integrate with his peers, but it is still amazing how many selfless children there are who we know. Hey, it's hard enough knowing who you are yourself in the fourth grade, but we have many great, patient, interesting kids who knock on the door and say "want to come out?" or "may I come in and see your room?" And then he's learning what can't be taught in school - friendship. Know this, too . . . God doesn't make any mistakes. David is perfect the way he is and, although my daily prayers are for "good days" and small successes, I've never prayed that he be NT or Neurotypical. We love him EXACTLY the way he is. God knew that He would have to choose a family with guts, strength, fortitude and love to take on the world - because some days, you will have to. I pity the small minds and nay-sayers who get in the way on those days. To take a line from Lynard Skynard, my favorite band, "you can hear me screaming a mile away" as I head toward the door.

July 12, 2012

Biopsy day. I'd be kidding if I said I hadn't wanted the day to both hurry up and get here and never get here. Sleep was non-existent, which also gave me extra time to tell myself not to worry until there was something to worry about and then to go ahead and worry anyway. Crazy-making.

I check into the Women's Breast Center and begin filling out the paperwork. I glance at the other patients who are there, too, trying to gauge their levels of anxiety or distress. Are they freaking out inside, despite the flipping through magazines and chatting? Is it just me? Are they here only for a check up and not invasive diagnostics? Can they tell that I am FREAKING OUT?

"Mrs. Minear, you can come on back," the nurse called brightly. "I don't want to," the irrational voice in my head said, "I want to run out of this room screaming!!!" I stand up and take my paperwork in with me to a little room to the left, with the standard gown open-in-the-back laying on the chair. The nurse questions a bit of background from me and a lot of background regarding finding the lump that is to be biopsied. I can tell nothing from her expression other than she does this a lot. How many women is "a lot"? She is neither rushed nor perfunctory in her questions, even though she doesn't need to look down to remember the next question. I feel "listened to", gaining comfort and resolve as I talk.

After she leaves, I gown up and wait to be called into the biopsy room, locking my belongings in the little locker and slipping the key to the locker tethered to a little bungie around my arm. There are a couple of other women there, in addition to my intake nurse, another nurse and a ultrasound technician. All smiling, encouraging, helping, caring, as I'm helped onto the table and made as comfortable as possible. The room is softly lit, but not dim, and the furnishings clean but not devoid of color, to soften the serious nature of what goes on in these four walls. Dr. Healer enters and the staff immediately stand a bit straighter in his presence. The good surgeon happens to be married to Dr. Joy, my Family Physician, and they are both the most professional, yet most personable doctors imaginable.

"Wow, your beard is really getting gray," I blurted, the nervous me kicking my already dented verbal filter clear off. The nurses thought that was hilarious . . . Dr. Healer, in mock dismay, reminded me to be nice to the Doctor who was going to be jabbing at me. I was helped onto my left side, right breast pointing (mostly) to the ceiling. A decade ago, it would have pointed skyward most certainly, but 38DDs have a habit of becoming less perky with age. Mine wasn't yet getting lost in my back-fat, but it was crowding my armpit.

Sliding the gown off of that side, Dr. Healer and company looked at the dimpled area. He pushed on it with his gloved fingers and was silent. "We're going to get some good samples of this thing so we know what we're dealing with. I'm going to numb you, which is really the worst of it. After you are numb, you may feel some pressure, but are really only going to hear some clicks like a ball-point pin. Although I can't feel anything in your armpit, I'll sample some nodes, too. That I can't really numb for." The ultrasound was going to be used to make sure that the team had a clear image of size and location of the lump, to make sure he had the best samples.

As the doctor imaged, pushed and clicked (6 times lump and 3 nodes), a warm hand held my right arm as it stretched over my head. "Click" Not holding in place or restraining, but the hand kept patting and rubbing, rubbing and patting, giving strength and comfort as I tried to be brave. "Click" I wasn't brave. On the inside, I wondered what kind of horror was inside me, unnamed but there taking up space in my body. The biopsy didn't seem real, like a nightmare, but with no monsters but the one within, and everyone holding me, patting me, soothing me was trying to keep the night terror at bay. "Click"

"Do you have kids?" one asked, to make conversation and to keep my mind off of the procedure. "Click" "Yes", I answered, "I have a big son from my husband's previous marriage. Billy's 24. And I have a nine year old named 'David'." I blurted "He has Aspergers, on the Autism Spectrum. He needs me, so I must live forever." "Click" And with that, the floodgates opened and tears rolled sideways off of my face and onto the table. No sobbing, just big, continuous tears that I couldn't control and didn't even care to. The warm hand on my arm rubbed and patted, patted and rubbed and the room fell silent. "Click"

After the biopsy was finished, I went back into the little room, opened the locker and retrieved my clothes and purse. The intake nurse gave me a two-inch bound book about breast cancer and treatments "in case the biopsy comes back positive" and said that Dr. Healer would talk to me in a few minutes. The 3 X 3 dressing on my right breast felt bulky, although I couldn't feel any discomfort. "I wonder if the tape is Latex-free", I thought, irrationally worrying about the tape welts my Latex sensitive body would produce if it was not.

Dr. Healer entered the room and sat down. Kindly, but not patronizingly, he said, "I think I know what this is. It looks like breast cancer to me."

He readjusted his position, leaning forward. "If it is, you have options," he said.

"You can have radiation to shrink it and a lumpectomy, Depending upon the pathology or the extent, you may have chemotherapy and radiation with a lumpectomy. You may decide to . . ."

I didn't give him a chance to finish. "Take them both."

He looked at me and repeated "Both?"

I answered as calmly as I could, "I'm not going through this again. I don't care if it is only one breast or that a lumpectomy would do. I need the most aggressive treatment I can get for my peace of mind. If it's cancer, take them both."

The good doctor gave a half-smile and a small nod, as if he understood and agreed. He then said, "well, this is Thursday and the biopsy results should be back on Tuesday. Let me get an appointment for you with a good plastic surgeon for reconstruction for Wednesday. If the results are negative, you can cancel the appointment. If positive, you can go in the next day and discuss reconstruction options." I protested that I wasn't going to have reconstruction if it was positive, as I wasn't going to go through anything else that wasn't absolutely necessary. Dr. Healer, nodded and gently suggested that I keep the appointment anyway and just *listen to the Plastics doctor. "You're still a young woman (at 44) and don't want to deal with prosthetics for the rest of your life, just think about it. You can have the expanders put in during the mastectomy and save yourself a surgery."*

I promised that I would, took my binder "just in case" and went home. I don't remember leaving, paying the parking attendant or driving home. I do remember pulling up to my house, realizing that I had been screaming for most of the way home. I walked into the kitchen, hugged Bill and sobbed while I recalled the appointment and my decision. I should have asked him before I made it, but I needn't have worried – double mastectomy was his vote, too.

July 17, 2012

Waiting is the worst part of treatment – maybe the second worst after actually receiving a diagnosis. As is my Type-A personality, I kept myself so busy that I couldn't dwell on my angst and fears during the days between biopsy and "D-Day" – "Diagnosis Day." That's only half-true. Just around the corner of full consciousness lurks the "what if" and the mantra "isitcancerisitcancerisitcancer" plays over and over like macabre background music.

For our son, we were determined to keep things as normal as possible. Bill and I took David to the pool in the evenings after work, even though my wounded biopsy-breast wouldn't allow me to get in. Man, the whole right side of my right breast was purple and red, before it began fading to green and red. I envisioned the good doctor, stabbing the monster over and over, killing it inside me. I also thought, if it is cancer, does a biopsy break any kind of sheath that a tumor is encapsulated in? Letting the cancer cells escape like a chick pecking its way out of an egg?

I couldn't control the wait (and I hate not being in control), but I could control my productivity during the wait. I cleaned closets and under the bed on the weekend. We visited Dad and Mino often during the weekend, running back and forth to their house. As Dad was recovering well from his brain surgery, we remained hopeful on his prognosis. Although we remained steeped in Faith, I wondered if God would have both Father and Daughter with different cancer diagnoses, six weeks apart. To question God is to accuse Him of being unjust, so not really questioning, but . . . what are the odds if it happened?

As for work, I'm strange in that one of my favorite hobbies is reading about and researching in my chosen field. I'm an oil and gas attorney – have been almost from the genesis of my career. With all the shale interest in Appalachia, <u>everyone</u> now claims to be an O & G attorney, but up until a very few years ago, there weren't many of us. For the days between biopsy and D-Day, I worked more than I usually work. Sleep was impossible, so I'd read old and new cases in my field or research the federal courts' dockets for acquisition strategies that other companies were using, perusing briefs the parties submitted to the courts for fun. On the day before D-Day, I travelled to the Pittsburgh area with colleagues to put on a presentation about compatible and divergent interests as to oil and gas versus coal. Although in the car during the drive home, we discussed a co-worker whose wife had been diagnosed with breast cancer, I didn't tell either one about my biopsy only a few days before – as if discussing it would jinx my results.

On July 17, I called the doctor's office five or six times, making sure they didn't miss pulling my results. "Nothing yet, Mrs. Minear," I was told, gently, "I promise we will call you the moment we have them." I couldn't stand not telling, so I did mention to a couple of friends at work that day. Walter, the Senior Paralegal, with whom I have worked the most and longest, was first. His beautiful wife had gone through early stage colon cancer in recent years and, not only does he "get it" from the trenches, he "gets" me, which is comforting. I also told Kathy, one of my absolute favorite people and who has a history of breast cancer in her family. Although Kathy works her project coordination magic in multiple states, she happened to be in Charleston for "D-Day."

Shortly after lunch (which I worked through), I called the doctor's office again. The same kind voice on the other end of the line didn't change, but she said, "Here it is, your results came in. They are positive. The tumor is Invasive Intraductal Carcinoma. I'm sorry. Had you decided on your course of care?"

I was in shock, I numbly told her that I had decided to undergo a double mastectomy and that I had an appointment with the plastic surgeon scheduled for the next day. She said, "Keep the appointment and we'll see if we can coordinate surgeries for the same time. It'll be alright."

I hung up the phone and went out of my office door, catching my arm on my purse as I did. In a daze walked down the open space of the office to the end of the hall, where my friend Kathy was in a meeting with another attorney and our internal clients, both in office and on the phone. I looked through the glass, caught her eye and gave her a small nod. She stood up and, with whomever on the conference call still talking, opened the door and wrapped me in the warmest hug . . . all five-foot nothing of her to five foot 10-inch me. I couldn't speak or I would have started to scream, but, as tears fell, I headed down the hall, down the elevators and across the parking lot to the van. Once inside, I wailed and screamed and pounded the inside of the car in anger and grief and fear. I screamed the whole way home, not caring that the other cars on the road would see this harpy in a gold minivan tearing at the inside of the vehicle, mouth wide in horror. In hindsight, I was probably too distraught to have driven – thank God for taking the wheel that afternoon.

Bill was working from home that day, so as soon as he heard me come through the door, he came upstairs from his basement office. I held it together (mostly) while relaying the news. I worried if he knew my level of distress it would make him feel more helpless than he already did, so I went upstairs to the bedroom to lie down, with him close behind. The Buddy came upstairs and played between us on the bed, while Bill and I held hands across the bed, not saying a word, each lost in our respective thoughts.

I Never Really Understood

When I was growing up, Dad was one of only two doctors in a really small town. I had been exposed to sickness and injury for most of my life. Whether it was a lawnmower accident or a classmate passing away from cancer not previously seen in someone so young, I was sympathetic, but not *empathetic* as I didn't really understand the depth and breadth of what was going on.

As an adult, and particularly an older adult, I experienced chronic illness from afar with co-workers, even helping some get their final affairs in order and cancer up close with one of my best friends. The latter, Mary Sue, was such a cool lady. When I work, it's not uncommon to see me either spread out on the floor or table, maps and plats and post-its all over the place, barefoot with a pencil in my hair as I lose myself in the task at hand. When Mary Sue worked, she'd get the same result, impeccably turned out in her suit and kick-ass shoes. I would tease her that she was appropriately named "Mary" after Mary Poppins as she was "practically perfect in every way".

Mary Sue passed away from colon cancer on Christmas Day 2008. Throughout her treatments, while she worked, I took my coffee into her office, which was next to mine, every morning, talking about work, family, trips (personal and business) and what was going on with her health and about coming to grips with David's challenges. When she went to the hospital with fevers during her treatments, she would call me to come over to keep her company, and we'd sit and talk . . . or not talk at all. I loved her husband, and delighted in stories about what her kids were doing (her son used to watch David) and I reassured her that she would beat her illness – but she didn't.

As close as I was to Mary Sue, my closest friend who had ever gone through treatment, and through her candor and her bravery, she could never have conveyed what it *feels* like to hear the word "carcinoma" attributed to yourself. Indescribable. What cancer has already given me is the empathy for others going through health issues, in addition to the sympathy that I've always felt. In my heart, I feel what is behind that look of fear and horror in the eyes of those with a cancer diagnosis. I know the angst behind the brave words and I know the worry and pain of those who love them.

I get it. And while I am constantly prayerful that no one else ever feels that awful "thud" in the pit of your stomach that accompanies the word "carcinoma", I know that, for now, that there will be others diagnosed with cancer. I pray it anyway. I also make sure to reach out to others either newly diagnosed or who have had cancer return to let them know that I know, and I GET IT, and that I continue to pray them through to peace.

July 18, 2012

A plastic surgeon's office is not where I thought I would ever be. Other than for disfiguring accidents, I relegated plastic surgery to those who wanted nipped, tucked, augmented, liposuctioned . . . to those who wanted to change themselves. I was perfectly happy (and remain so) with my too-large nose and mouth, large pores, sun spots, muffin-top and under-eye luggage (not bags, but full luggage). Through the years, I had considered a breast reduction, as 38DDs are not comfortable and hard to fit into clothes, but anesthesia is not to take lightly, so the thoughts were fleeting. God has a sense of humor and let me have breast reduction the hard way.

As David's sitter, Sarah, was on vacation with her family, Bill stayed home to watch David while I went to the consultation alone. The waiting room I walked into was not what I expected. Instead of seeing a roomful of teased primped and heavily-made up women (there was one of those) the patients were men and women, a few with clear hand or arm injuries, and one woman with a pretty scarf over her bald head. I was immediately at ease and hopeful and more than a little ashamed at myself for pre-judging (yes, God, I'm working on it).

I filled out the intake information – again – and waited. Shortly, I was called back through the door to the far back of the office and a cozy, comforting consultation room with a 3-angle mirror, vanity table with a computer and shelves of breast implants arranged as if in a gift shop. Some were under glass and they were all morbidly fascinating to me.

The nurse took a little more information and said that the doctor would be in soon. Dr. Healer had recommended Dr. Bulldog and I was grateful that he had a slot for consultation available so soon for me. Admittedly, I was a little apprehensive to see what he looked like . . . the "judgmental me" thought "if he looks like a Ken-doll, I'm out of here." I didn't want someone with 90210 expectations of what he was going to do for me – 25314 is just fine. When Dr. Bulldog walked in and introduced himself, I was relieved. He's a very nice looking man, but not pinched, pulled or tweaked-looking. He even had some gray in his curly hair.

The doctor booted the computer and started a video about what to expect with reconstruction after mastectomy and some of the procedures available. He and the nurse left the room to while I watched, promising to return afterward for discussion and questions. The video was computer graphic generated, largely, showing different techniques. When it was finished, I was also able to view some "before and after" photos of women (headless, nameless photos) who had similar procedures. I still wasn't convinced that I wanted to reconstruct, but the thought of prostheses for the rest of my life was a worse image so I listened.

Then the dreaded part . . . Dr. Bulldog needed to look at my breasts to get some ideas and recommend, so, during the video, I had put on the standard patient gown. Pre-cancer, I wouldn't have been self-conscious. Now, however, as I hadn't looked down at my lumped, biopsied self since I found the lump, the thought of someone else glimpsing offending breast made me ill. I worried (irrationally) that he could see the evil lurking just below the surface and would recoil at the sight – or that, like in the movie "Alien", it would shoot out and rip his hand off.

As with any situation where I feel uncomfortable, I make jokes. As he was measuring left and right, from the navel and from the shoulder, from each other and what-not, I wondered out loud that I had always wanted to get back on the stripper pole that got me through law school and, if he could see fit to make me double-Gs after surgery I could quit law and "ride the pole again." He blinked . . . and smiled. My kind of doctor – twisted humor. As Dr. Bulldog finished, took photos and wrapped the gown around me again, he brought out an expander and let me hold it. Hard, egg-shaped, but flat, he explained that, if I elect to do both surgeries at the same time, after the surgeon finished with the mastectomy, he would insert the expanders under the muscle and skin. Otherwise, I could come back for another surgery and he'd insert the expanders, it was my call.

Either way, every couple of weeks or so, I would come in and he would fill the expanders little by little until we got the size I was comfortable with. Dr. Bulldog asked me if I had an idea of what size. I said that I'd be happy with a full "C" – although I'm a big woman, I had no desire to get near the Ds again, even if it messed with my proportions. He slid the equivalent implant off of the shelf and let me touch and hold it while explaining that, after I had expanded to the right size, he'd switch out the expanders and insert the implants. We also discussed (and I quickly rejected the "flap procedure" options. With a flap, they take muscle and tissue from another part of your body and, leaving the blood vessels connected, transplant to the breast area. Most flaps are from the lower abdomen or scapula area. Maybe in the future, but planning additional surgeries at that point was not what I wanted. Also, it's slightly alarming to me to think that I could scratch my chest and have my brain register "back".

As I left, his nurse promised to coordinate some dates with Dr. Healer's schedule to see if we could get it set soon. The reality of diagnosis, surgeries, appointments, etc., hadn't truly set in yet, so I was glad to be moved along, told and shown the next step, surrendering control to those who could help get me through. I'm no shrinking violet and my husband a former paramedic, but I think we were both in shock and trusting those healthcare professionals could get us where we needed to be when we had the faculties to take my care back over. When to have surgery, how extensive the surgery, who would stay with the Buddy, start reconstruction now or later, who will be the oncologist, what will the tests say about staging, will I need chemotherapy, what about radiation . . .? All of this without knowing my precise diagnosis and prognosis and on top of worrying about my projects, clients, workload, co-workers, etc. – "yes", I know those thoughts should be secondary, but I've been Type-A for so long, even cancer needs to get in the queue.

What I Don't Know Scares Me

The shock of breast cancer, or any cancer, is terror-inducing. Knowing that you have been invaded by an enemy whose very name is often whispered is nauseating. For me, the words "breast cancer" at least called its name out loud – and solved some of the question of why I'd been so dog-assed tired for so long. Like getting a diagnosis for my son's Asperger's, knowledge is power. I can fight what I know, plan for what I know . . . it's the unknown that scares the hell out of me.

For perspective, and as I've mentioned, one of my best friends passed away in 2008. Mary Sue was diagnosed with breast cancer in 2006 and had a single mastectomy in July of that year, followed by radiation. Her body was healing from the surgery, but she wasn't feeling better. Follow-up testing in October 2006 revealed that, while she was being treated for early-stage breast cancer, she also had unrelated, Stage 4 colon cancer. It wasn't the cancer she knew of originally that ultimately led to her passing.

I was afraid, yes, of the breast cancer, but my fears compounded with my experience with one of my dearest friends. Both oil and gas attorneys, offices side-by-side, she 46 at first diagnosis, me at 44 and breast cancer our first diagnosis . . . Would another cancer follow for me as well?

In coordinating dates between the offices for my mastectomies and reconstruction, we settled on July 26, 2012, that would work for both doctors. Actually, the coordination was odd . . . it was, "well, you can do July 26, August 8 or August 22 . . ." *Are you kidding!?!* I know I should have seen it as a positive that they were so convinced it wouldn't progress in that time that it wasn't a "tomorrow" surgery, like for my friend. It was unthinkable for me to wait. Toward the days leading up to the surgery, I seriously contemplated taking my husband's hack saw and hacking my right breast off myself. What stopped me is that, in our filled-to-the-brim garage, it would have taken me until late August to find the saw. I wanted the damn thing off and out NOW. I swear I could feel the cancer creeping toward my lymph nodes. I took July 26th.

In the eight *long* days between diagnosis and surgery, the fear of the unknown cancer lurking elsewhere in my body consumed me. When confirming the surgery for the 26th, I trusted Dr. Healer's gal Friday, with my fear of the unknown. She is actually "Friday" and the other six days of the week for that office, all while exuding a warmth and kindness that invites such trust. Friday managed to work an MRI appointment in for me on Friday, July 20th.

While at the MRI, filling out the dreaded paperwork, I scanned the room, trying to figure out what the others were there for. Trying to hear, but to *not* overheard conversations. Some were impossible to not overheard. Some folks have the amazing ability to talk loudly and openly about the most graphic details of their affliction or, embarrassingly, that of their loved-one or friend who is back in Imaging, oblivious that the waiting room has heard their colon polyp count as of the last appointment. I am open with my diagnosis, but will never be able to muster such a casual discussion about it. Cancer is formal, to me, to be respected, not casual.

Back in the MRI, the lady technician had me gowned and prepped, asked the same questions as to diagnosis, location, etc.

and inserted an intravenous line. Although I drank the trough of radioactive contrast before the appointment, I was also having the IV contrast as well. Thank God, the tech told me that, when she would start the IV contrast, it would feel as if I needed to go to the bathroom, but, not to panic, as I really didn't have to go. The MRI would take about 20 minutes.

As soon as the lights dimmed and she went into the booth to start the equipment, I began to cry quietly, arms over my head, machine whirling. Wondering if I would be lighting up the scans with these horrible, murderous tumors all over my body in addition to the one that I knew. Wondering if she could see the cancer in my right breast, if it looked stranger still with the six biopsy punctures. Wondering how many others would file through Imaging that day, or any day, faced with the same horror that accompanied my tears and the whir of the MRI that day. And she was right, "starting the IV contrast" she said, and immediately my bladder started to feel warm and I thought, "I wonder how many others would pee on her table today" for I was sure I was going to.

After I finished, I was told that the doctors would read my scans and let me know if there was anything else by the following Tuesday. Four long days away. Thankfully, I had a lot to keep me busy. In 2012 and 2013, I Chaired the Legal group of a multi-discipline natural gas association. That meant that I was scheduled to be in Fort Worth, Texas, on the Monday through the Wednesday before my Thursday surgery. I had debated with Bill about whether I should go or not . . . I really wanted to spend as much time with him and David as I could, while I was still in the same shape. Bill urged me to go, both since I had worked so hard on getting the conference together (and I really enjoy my field of law and my colleagues at other companies) and since time passes more quickly when you are busy. No doubt I needed the distraction – doubly-so as I waited for the MRI results.

In hind-sight, I can't believe I went. On two days before surgery, while in Texas, as I called Friday at Dr. Healer's office, it dawned on me the magnitude of being so far away. What happened if, as my greatest fear, the results were that I did have other hot spots on my body, other than the breast cancer? If that were the case, midway through the full day of the conference, I would fall apart. I would cease to function. How would I ever be able to pack to get back on the airplane and get home? Would Bill and David need to come and get me, another colleague, a friend or would someone from the conference need to get me together and get me to the airport? I really hadn't thought through my being half the country away and waiting for test results.

Thankfully, when I called (and had Bill call, too, to confirm) I was told that the MRI showed nothing else. "Just breast cancer?" I asked – naming the beast that I knew and was reassured that there wasn't also an unknown beast that I didn't. Although I still had breast cancer, and was two days from being "Beth after mastectomy" I spent the remainder of the conference in sheer elation, with one of my greatest fears being beaten down. "Elation" at "just cancer" is an oxymoron, I know, but turning the T-Rex back into a crocodile was comforting.

I flew home a morning early from the conference, as I had my final Plastic Surgery appointment on the day before the mastectomies. I was getting my "before and after" breasts photographed. Dr. Bulldog drew the symmetry lines on my chest with purple marker from just under the hollow in my throat to the top of my navel, giving himself a roadmap during surgery to begin reconstruction so that the reconstruction would be even, top to bottom, left to right. It definitely showed above my black and white blouse (and I was heading to the grocery afterward), but the markings, to me, were a comforting, tangible step to getting the cancer removed – no hack saw required.

The Telling

Telling friends and co-workers about my diagnosis and decision to have the double mastectomy was relatively simple. I've always been an open book about David's Asperger's, believing that, with being open, we may be able to save other families and kids the angst and mistakes made, by us and others, in navigating the diagnosis, therapy, school, treatment, IEP mazes. I treat breast cancer the same way – Bill does, too. Although I caution him that having breast cancer doesn't mean everything is free game. Revealing my occasional constipation is in no way relevant to the cancer conversation and I didn't waive the right to keep private what I can when I became a patient. And I am *very* private in general – I don't even have a Facebook, because what I want people to know, I tell them personally.

I told Dad and Mino first, largely because, as I try to support and back Mino up in caring for Dad as much as possible, I would be out of commission for the next few weeks after surgery, so would be less help. God Bless my Dad, as tired as he still was seven weeks after brain surgery, and through tough tears, he assured my "you're going to be fine, I know it." I agreed and said he was going to be, too, and he smiled and nodded. Mino cried and worried and sent up prayers.

Telling my Mother was tough. Although we had enjoyed a nearly-perfect relationship until the past couple of years, we were estranged recently by disappointments in each other. Now, I think God gave this buffer to us so we could handle my diagnosis with the other. Tough, too, is that she and I have never valued looks the same. She worries about hair, makeup, clothing, etc. and I've always frustrated her that these are not important to me. Should I put a little more effort in my appearance? Probably. My standard "uniform" is black, black and white, tan or other neutrals and hair usually up in a clip. So I wasn't surprised when Mother asked "Do you need to do that? Did you get a second opinion?" I assured her that I was comfortable with my decision, as was Bill, that they are called "boobs" for a reason, as they are just "boobs", and I had already nursed my son. I did ask her to tell my sister, who was on vacation, but to wait until they came back so to not ruin her time. When we hung up, I could tell that she was working through . . . processing the information, but, to her credit, she held it together on the phone. She held it together for me, knowing that I'm uncomfortable with overly emotional displays – for her strength during that call, I'm grateful.

Bill and I did not tell and, as of this writing, still have not told our David about Mom having cancer. He was a new nine when I was diagnosed and we believe in letting a kid be as free of adult worries as they can. Our son will spend the vast majority of his life as an adult and needs to be able to focus on his Aspie "fascinations" and not worry about his Mommom. He knows "surgery" but not cancer.

We did tell my stepson (hate that word), Billy, and Bill's Mom and Dad. Billy rose to the occasion, pledged support and love for whatever we needed and has been Bill's rock. Our son, David, is named after Bill's younger brother, Dave, who died of cancer at age 38 back in 1996, leaving behind my two nieces at a young age. Bill and Dave were 17 months apart and inseparable growing up. We handled Bill's parents carefully, as both were in their late 80s and had already lost Dave to cancer. When I became pregnant with David, our deal was that if it was a girl, I'd name the baby and Bill would if it was a boy. When the ultrasound revealed David's gender, Bill immediately named him after his brother. Mom and Dad Minear took the news with the love, strength and dignity that they display every day. I do know, from conversations, that their worry for me is touched and magnified by their loss of Dave.

The one friend I was anxious to tell was also on vacation during my diagnosis week. While Deanna is one of my newest friends (only six years at the time of diagnosis) she is definitely one of my best. Although she is much better than I at keeping up with getting her hair done and clothing up to date, Deanna is no fluff – my girl is *definitely* substance over form and the most like me of any friend. I knew I'd need her strength and substantial fortitude to get me through this . . . to get US through this.

Deanna, unfortunately, had recent experience with what I was facing. Her best friend, Donna, who I had only heard stories about (hilarious), but hadn't yet met, had been diagnosed with breast cancer the year before, had also chosen a double mastectomy and had been six months or so finished with treatment. Besides being "Deanna", and the most together person I know, she had been through the fire with Donna and could bring that to bear.

I was right in my assessment – on the Sunday after she came back from vacation, and five days before my surgery, I left a message on her voice-mail to get back to me. Bill and I were with the Buddy at a playground when my phone rang. It was Deanna. We talked about her vacation, and work and when Sarah (who had watched David in the summers for years) would be available – normal conversation. We paused and, as I draped myself over the slide (Bill had moved the Buddy out of ear-shot), I told Deanna that I had breast cancer, that surgery was next week and that we may need a little extra help.

There was none of the pitying words, no sign of "tut-tut" in her voice that had always made me cringe, and not just when I told folks that the Buddy had Asperger's. True to her personality, she said, "well, let's put on your big girl panties and get ready to kick some ass." Immediately, as I knew she would . . . as I had *hoped* she would, she took over. Deanna began planning the week, the surgery, the recovery, wrangling David, giving Bill a break . . . she took over everything so I could focus just on me. My friend, with the greatest imposition, the greatest favor I had ever asked of anyone, rose to the challenge and pole-vaulted over the impossibly high bar, without hesitation. She commandeered her amazing family, as well, declared them to be "Team Beth" for whatever we needed, whenever we needed and truly carried our family into the light beyond the tunnel of my surgery with strength, humor and Faith.

July 26, 2012

"I haven't slept all night," I thought. I'm wide awake at 4:30 a.m., apprehensive, but anxious to get on with it. The only other surgery I'd had to date is the C-section to deliver David who was frank breech at birth. From that blessed occasion to this one . . . I could tell that Bill was awake, too. He had taken his CPAP off (it took me nine years to convince him he had sleep apnea) and was quietly lying next to me. Sensing that I was awake as well, Bill reached over and grasped my hand, saying nothing. There was nothing to say.

"Go downstairs and start your coffee," I whispered, not wanting to wake up David who was sleeping in Billy's bedroom. "Have some breakfast for me, too." I wasn't allowed to eat anything before surgery and hadn't since the night before. "What time is Sarah getting here?" he asked. "She'll be here by 8:00," I answered, "plenty of time before the 8:30 check in." As surgery isn't scheduled until 11:00, I knew we had time to spare even from that. David will wake up and Sarah will be here. Not Mom. He knows Mom is having surgery, but his relation to "surgery" is when the dentist put him to sleep for his "pirate tooth", so he's not worried. And Sarah is one of his favorite people in the world. Not Mom, but pretty damn close.

Bill moves downstairs to start his routine, paper, coffee, breakfast, Blackberry . . . I am grateful for the routine. Despite our world being upside-down, routine helps keep everyone feeling normal. I flip on the bedside light and get out of bed, walking to the guestroom to check my overnight bag. "What exactly do you pack for a double-mastectomy?" I wondered. I had been told to get loose-fitting shirts that button up, as I'll be heavily bandaged and won't be able to put my arms up to wear pull-on shirts. None of my wardrobe fit the bill, but my Bill's did – he of the "Tommy Bahama" Hawaiian shirts. I had packed a couple of his largest and softest shirts in my bag, along with random odds and ends (cotton swabs, tea bags, lotion, hair clip, toothbrush). I had also packed a small devotional book and a notebook with which to jot random thoughts as I had them . . . and which chronicles have lent themselves to this book. These had been sent to me by a Mother from Philadelphia whose son also has Asperger's. We've never met, but Becky is part of my Twitterverse of Mother Warriors of children on the Autism Spectrum – a woman of great Faith and fortitude, sending her support and prayers. We share triumphs, meltdowns, frustrations at the neuro-typical world and its barriers and aspects of our lives that we would share with in-the-flesh friends. Mother's of special needs children generally have unending fortitude, resources and Faith and I needed my Mother Warriors to put those vibes into action for my sake this time, not just my son's.

I zipped up the overnight bag for the hundredth time and walked it downstairs to the front of the door. I checked the contents of the refrigerator, having stocked it the day with David's favorite foods – pudding, fruit, applesauce, water bags, green beans, corn, yoghurt, cheese - as well as cooking a vat of spaghetti that should carry him and us through the weekend. The insurance company has a mastectomy listed as a one-day stay, so I should be home by tomorrow, Friday afternoon, if all goes well. Drive-through amputations, at your service.

I went back upstairs and ran a hot bath, slipping into it for a long soak. I prefer baths, not showers, and knew that this would be my last of either for a few weeks or at least until the incisions had healed enough that I wouldn't risk infection. Lying in the tub, I tried not to look down at the still-bruised biopsy site. Surreal experience, knowing that you wake up with body parts and will end the day without them. "What do they do with them?" I wondered, envisioning rows and rows of shelves in the basement of the hospital and a place in the "Boob Section" with a slot neatly labeled "MINEAR X2".

I did the "lather, rinse, repeat" on my hair, shaved my legs, pumiced my feet, spending all my energy focusing on the task at hand, tucking the horror of what lay before me – before US – to the back of my mind. After 40 minutes or so, I got out, toweled off and dressed in stretch jeans and top. I hadn't packed additional pants, so I wore what was comfortable enough for me to come home in the following day.

A few hours later, Sarah showed up (early) and, although she's watched the Buddy for years, followed me on her crutches around the first floor, letting me show her again where everything was and what was in the fridge. Sarah had broken her ankle playing softball (and was on scholarship at a University in another state), but never complained. I think she knew I needed to, to "Mother" my son while he slept upstairs, oblivious to the drama below him. She quietly assured me that they'd be fine, wished me well and closed and locked the door behind us as we headed for the hospital. "God, watch over my son," I prayed, "and don't give him a moment of distress about his Mommom." As we pulled away from our home, with me intact for the last time, I was hit by a wall of sadness so profound, that it left me too wounded to even cry. Bill did enough for both of us.

Checking into surgery prep, I am amazed at the clinical ballet that unfolds. Patient names on wallboards, clip boards and beds, doctor's and nurses' names beside in neat squares. Gowns donned, IVs started, vitals taken . . . all smoothly, seamlessly coordinated for the minimum of confusion and efficiency.

A crisp, but kind nurse takes charge of getting me settled and goes back to get Bill from the waiting room where he'd been since dropping me off and parking the car. I wanted to call her back, to tell her that this awful game had gone on long enough and that I didn't want to play anymore. It couldn't be real, right? Three weeks and one day ago I found and lump and now I'm having my breasts amputated. Did I make the right decision? I'm pretty sure there is no "do-over" if I change my mind after the surgery. That thought was fleeting, as I knew that I had to take the most-aggressive action that I could to beat this cancer – that I would remove every body part if I meant that I could stay with my family and help my son reach his potential.

Bill came in and sat next to the chair where I now sat bare-butted, my clothes in the plastic bag that hospitals give you for procedures. The 38DD bra that I would never wear again (or any of its sisters) and my underwear tucked into the toes of my shoes so they wouldn't show through the plastic bag. I had brought my Blackberry and kept working, keeping my mind occupied, getting as much as I could off of my desk and kicked back to my clients until I could pick matters back up. I had quit my private practice six years prior, when the Buddy had been diagnosed, and had come in-house to the gas company which, at the time, had been my biggest client. Although we lost about 2/3 of my annual income coming in-house, having back-up during the years we were getting my son on track and now knowing that I had coverage for my cases during this surgery more than made up for it.

"In here," the nurse said to the orderly, who had come with the gurney to wheel me back to the holding area before surgery. I climbed on the bed, taking care to keep the gown closed across my middle-aged rump. "Good luck" she said, and "you'll do fine", as I know was the routine, and I was wheeled away. The orderly drove my hospital bed around corners and into the elevator more smoothly than I drive our van. He kept a light banter with Bill, not asking too many questions or letting the conversation slip, playing his role in patient care with great kindness. Dropping me off in my designated slot in the curtained waiting area, Bill and I thanked him – he smiled, patted my covered foot and went back out the door.

A beautiful woman, gowned and smiling, came over to my bed, checked my chart and said "Hi, I'm the Nurse Anesthetist who will be assisting the Anesthesiologist during your surgery today. When was the last time you had anything to eat? Would you please open your mouth so I can look at your airway? Any dentures or partials? Any prior problems with anesthesia?" I answered, opened my mouth, shook my head and she dutifully jotted my responses. "I see you have Dr. Healer today," she beamed. "We all love working with him." Bill and I confessed that we felt really fortunate to have him, too. There are some great surgeons in the Kanawha Valley, but I feel certain that none are better". I normally eschew small talk, but her words were welcome and comforting.

An older doctor came over to my bed, greeted the Nurse Anesthetist and introduced himself "I'm your Anesthesiologist today. When was the last time you had anything to eat? Would you please open your mouth so I can look at your airway? Any dentures or partials? Any prior problems with anesthesia?" Again, I answered, opened my mouth and shook my head. "Good, good." He said. "As soon as Dr. Healer talks to you and gives us the go-ahead, we'll get started."

As both the Anesthesiologist and Nurse Anesthetist moved off, Bill and I saw Dr. Healer enter the holding room. He immediately came over to the side of the bed, shook hands with Bill, who he hadn't seen since Bill's colonoscopy a few years back and went through the basics of the procedure – enough so that we knew what to expect, but not too much so that we'd freak. He told Bill that they'd take him to the waiting room, where my sister would also be waiting, after they wheeled me back, and that the entire surgery, from the mastectomy through when Dr. Bulldog takes over midway to insert the expanders, would take approximately six hours. The doctor asked if either of us had any questions. Neither did. Bill thanked him, as did I.

Dr. Healer took my hand in both of his, looked me in the eye and said "God has both of us for this."

At that, the emotions that I tried so desperately to keep in check came flooding through. Not only the horror of reality, but the relief that comes from being in the hands of a doctor who, skilled as he is, knows who is really in control. No M.D.iety, is Dr. Healer, but a man of Faith in whom we put our trust and faith, while yielding to God's ultimate wisdom and grace. I sobbed as he squeezed my hand and headed out to the surgery room. My big, sweet husband, sobbing as well, kissed me and said "I love you. I'll be waiting." I could still hear him crying as they wheeled me back to surgery.

I didn't remember being in a surgery room like this when I had David. That had been more of a large suite and although it had bright lights and equipment, I didn't remember it looking so intimidating, so cold. Of course, that surgery was such a joyous occasion, I wouldn't have noticed if it was on the floor of a cave. The surgical team who were already in the room and in place, maneuvered me from the gurney onto the surgery table with a well-coordinates slide from one to the other. A large, truly alien-looking circular light hung from the ceiling. I could hear the conversations around me, but couldn't focus on anyone. "OhmyGod, this is really happening" I thought, trying as I had for the past three weeks, with varying success, not to scream. Tears kept flowing on both sides of my face, but my arms were tugged to the sides as a disembodied hand placed a mask over my nose and mouth, so I couldn't wipe them away. I didn't care, anyway. I could see reflections and movement in the stainless surface of the light above my head, but couldn't discern who was moving or what was going on. "This room is freezing," I thought . . .

* *

Waking, waking, sound, light, itching, aching. There is a vise around my chest and my tongue is dry and thick. Waking up in recovery is scary. Still largely immobile from the IV, the pain medication, catheter, pressure socks on my legs hooked to a machine to prevent clots, blood-pressure cuff . . . in recovery to be monitored and looked after, yet the only thing I needed was emotional. "Is my husband here?" I asked. No one looked over or up. Did I say it out loud? Could anyone hear me? Morphine makes me so itchy – I tried to scratch my arms, but couldn't move them to scratch. 'Don't panic", I thought, "your brain is awake, but the rest of you hasn't caught up."

Listening to the conversations, switching between summer talk and medicine – soothing is the normalcy in this abnormal room. Opening my eyes and keeping them open is a chore, but it gets me to Bill. A recovery nurse, smart in her blues, notices that I'm back from inner-space and smiles. She makes soothing noises, nonsensical chatter, while checking my vitals, my eyes, the four drains, two on each side of my torso, the pulse in my feet and I am comforted by her attention. "Is my husband here", I ask, again, confident that she can hear me. She smiles, "in the waiting room. Dr. Healer talked to him after the first part of your surgery a few hours ago and Dr. Bulldog did a short while ago. You did fine. We've told your husband you are waking up and we'll get him as soon as we can." The nurse took my temperature, checked the IV and gave me some ice chips, resuming the soothing sounds and nonsensical chatter.

I wondered what time it was – no clock was visible. Sarah was watching the Buddy for the first part of the day, my Mother taking over in late afternoon and then Bill in the evening. Deanna volunteered to stay with me in the hospital at night so Bill could go home, get some rest and let the Buddy sleep in our bed with him, to keep him reassured and comforted. All children are comforted by routine – those on the Autism Spectrum are especially sensitive to large upheavals (even some small ones). I knew that I could only focus on healing if I knew David was all right.

I heard Bill before I saw him, his big voice and big personality fill a room, charming everyone. Then his handsome face – so tired, so worried, so happy to see me came into focus. I'm sure I look like shit and smell like hospital funk, but he leans over and gives me the best kiss (fine, second best to our first kiss). I don't remember much about the conversation, checking in with each other emotionally. I ask the time and about David. Bill said, "It's a little after 7:30. You were under almost seven hours." It felt like only a flash. "David is with Wham (my Mother) and getting lots of attention. Deanna will be here around 9:00, but I want to get you settled into your room before I go."

As if on cue, my nurse came over, rechecked my IV, vitals, pulse, drains temperature and said that the ward was nearly full, but that they had a bed for me in a double until a private room opened up. Honestly, I didn't care. If the whoosh of the leg squeezers didn't bother her, it didn't bother me – at least tonight. I knew I'd sleep tonight (as well as you can in a hospital) so my roommate would need to be some kind of interesting to keep me awake.

At nearly 8:30, I am discharged from recovery to the main hospital ward. It's hard to get your bearings, full of morphine, bodies on either side of you, glimpsing mostly ceiling and wall-tops and I snooze off and on during the short trip. Double room – tiny, tiny – small bathroom, flimsy curtain between the beds. Deanna has come early (I knew she would) to help me get settled. She and Bill have an easy, familiar banter – giving each other support and crap at the same time. "You look good," she lies, and she knows that I know she's lying, but that's the game. Deanna gives me the highlights from Sarah's reports on David, well-wishes from the office (she's worked all day) and my elderly roommate in the next bed fills in the gaps. We're talking quietly, but her shadow is pressed against the curtain – she's enjoying being a part of.

Deanna has done the "girlfriend-with-mastectomy" routine before – in the hospital with her best friend (and now my dear friend) Donna. She stayed with Donna in the hospital, too, and knows more about what to expect that Bill or me. From the emotional to the physical, I'm in good hands, as was Donna before me.

"Go take care of the Buddy," I nudge Bill. "Tell him his Mommom is doing fine and misses him." I can tell it's hard for Bill to leave me, but he knows that what is best for me is taking care of our son and getting rest so he can take over from Deanna in the morning. Deanna lovingly, but firmly bustles him out of the room and makes her nest between my bed and the wall on the fold-out chair that turns into a half bed. A male nurse comes in and asks me to rate my pain between 1 and 10. "It's a "4" but that's fine," I answer. "You know, Morphine doesn't work well for me and makes me itchy. Percocet was what worked when I had my C-section." The nurse assures me that Morphine is stronger than Percocet and will keep me comfortable.

* *

White hot pain, vise around my chest has turned into a flame-thrower . . . unbearable, inescapable, indescribable. "Deanna," I croak, knowing I won't be able to muster more. She's up immediately, rolling off the make-shift bed. "Pain?" she asks, and I nod, movement hurting more. She zips down the hall, not waiting to push the button and wait for a response. In a minute, the nurse comes into the room. "Rate your pain, please," he asks. "Nine-plus," I whisper, as the Morphine goes into the IV and takes the edge off.

The nurse checks vitals, urine output, temperature, pulses in my feet while Deanna goes gets a drink and goes to the bathroom. We've awakened my roommate, who scampers into the bathroom as soon as Deanna leaves it. The nurse goes back down the hall. My roommate exits the bathroom, but continues to break-wind as she heads back to her bed. As sore as I am and as tired as Deanna has got to be, we giggle like 4th Graders at Ms. Flatulence in the next bed and we settle back in.

* *

"Here we go again," I think, flame thrower back in action. This time, I didn't need to say a word – Deanna is awake and out the door in an instant. A different nurse this time, young woman, brisk, careful. "Can you rate your pain?" she asks. "Nine-plus," I answer. "Percocet has generally worked better for me than Morphine." She injects the Morphine into the IV, and says "Morphine is supposed to be better than Percocet, but some meds work better than others on different people. I'll see if we can get orders for Percocet the next time around." She gives me a drink of water while my roommate, who we've again awakened, dashes into the bathroom, apparently afraid that Deanna will beat her to it.

My new nurse leaves as I ask Deanna what time it is. "Almost 6:00," she answers, "the last round was around 1:00." She moves toward the bathroom as my roommate emerges. In the semi-darkness, she looks at me and stops Deanna, "what's wrong with her?" she asks in a stage-whisper. Deanna tells her and I can see *my roomie trying to peer through the darkness at me. I keep my eyes slitted so I can watch her, watching me as Deanna closes the bathroom door. In a minute, she loses interest and gets back into her own bed. Deanna gets back onto her rack, we giggle again at my roommate and try to catch some sleep.*

July 27, 2012

Fully Friday now . . . I see Deanna going back into the bathroom to freshen up for the day, beating out my roommate who is oblivious and snoring loudly in the next bed. Bill will be here soon, Sarah watching David, and Deanna will head into work to start her workday. God Bless her.

Morning shift nurses check vitals and bodily functions while food trays are distributed. Bill and Deanna trade off, as mine is set on the bedside table. "If we can get your pain under control with oral medication, not IV, and for you to eat something, you'll be discharged today." Bill looked over at me – "Rough night?" he asked. "Brutal, but better now." I answered. "Rate your pain, please," the morning nurse asks. ""Four" I respond, and mention to see if they have the orders for Percocet. "Not yet," she chirps, "but we won't see the doctor until later this morning. You have a prescription of Dilaudid – we'll give you that to stay ahead of the pain."

"What's that," I ask. "Morphine-like" the nurse responded. "Morphine doesn't work well for me," I say "only Oxycodone . . . Percocet . . . works well for me" She smiles, that "I know better than you" smile that some healthcare folks plaster on, "Dilaudid is stronger. If we can get you to tolerate oral pain relief and some food, you can go home today." I'm too tired to go through it again – thankful that I'm only a "4", but knowing I'll be a "9" on the Morphine before it's time for another dose. I hope they can find a doctor to write a Percocet prescription for me.

Another nurse, young male, pops his head in and says that they are discharging another patient and would I still like a private room? As if on cue, Deanna pops her head out of the bathroom, hair fixed and face on and answered for me "Yes, we would." She packs her things away and begins to pack mine – ready the moment we can move. Less than an hour later, they have my catheter bag laying on my legs, IV being carried and wires to the monitors on the sides of my shoulders. I'm being wheeled away from my room, looking at the ceiling and wall-tops again, Deanna by my side, directing movement. It looks like we've gone down the hall, around the nurses' station and up another hallway. "I don't even know what floor I'm on," I think, not that it matters.

"Much better," Deanna announces, as we enter my new room. She's right . . . it's a small private, but a better layout – and quiet. No snoring or farting can be heard. "Would you make sure Bill knows my new room number?" I ask. "I've already texted him. He's parking the car," Deanna answered, as the nurses reconnect me to the monitors and scoot me up on the bed (I'm a butt-walker, working my way toward my toes)." A few minutes later, my sweet husband walks in, looking much better than yesterday.

"How's the Buddy?" I ask, accepting his tender kiss. "Great . . . still sleeping," he answers, and fills me in on the previous night at home. We then fill him in on my funny roommate and he laughs. "O.K.," Deanna announces, "I'm going to work. Let me know if you need anything. If they keep you another night, let me know and I'll stay." She gives him a brief overview of my pain medication situation and heads out.

"Thanks, Helga," Bill says.

"You're welcome, Hop-Sing," she responds with a huge smile as she disappears.

"What's all that?" I ask.

"She's 'Nurse Helga' for you and I'm 'Hop-Sing' like on "Bonanza", keeping the Homestead going." Hilarious – and so their personalities together. I drift off to sleep as they bring the breakfast tray in. I'm still not hungry so I leave it to Bill to eat, escaping the dull throb in my chest and pinch of IV line to sleep. I awaken again shortly before mid-day (no concept of actual time) as I can feel the torch being lit on the flame thrower. Not full-blown agony yet, but on its way. I look over to Bill, thumbing his Blackberry and croak "honey . . . can you check on meds? I'd really like to get in front of this." He hops up and heads to the nurses' station. We don't use the call-button if we can avoid it. We can get up and ask for help and it must be annoying for the nurses to hear that beep all day.

The young male nurse comes in, "it's not time yet for another dose, hon. I'm sorry. Can you rate your pain?" I close my eyes, "a 7, but moving. Can you do an Ibuprofen? IV, if you can. My stomach is empty and it kills me on an empty stomach." He did and in a few minutes the pain nudged down a bit to "not screaming, but bearable." I still wasn't hungry when they brought the lunch tray in, so Bill munched on some. I can't eat when I hurt. This continued for the rest of the day. Pain would spike, they'd give me Dilaudid, not crushing the pain and wearing off too soon – I'd sleep when I could, sipping water when I was awake. "Nurse Helga" texted "Hop-Sing" from time to time, checking on her patient.

My sister came to relieve Bill in late afternoon, so he could be with the Buddy and Sarah could go home. Deanna came in the early evening. I was awake enough to tease her that she really just wanted to not miss any action. As my sister lives out of town, she gave words of encouragement and started for home. I was grateful, but not surprised that she and my mother slide into the rotation without being asked.

The afternoon shift nurse was a pretty, spunky, 30is lady. She chatted a little bit as she checked vitals and gave me pain meds, saying that Dr. Healer was going to be in to check on me (and had the day before, but I didn't remember). Although the Dilaudid doesn't work well, it does wipe me out. I drifted off and barely remember Dr. Healer coming in that evening. Deanna filled me in. She said that he took my hand and asked "are you too mad at me?" knowing the pain I was in. She said that I had told him "no" and thanked him. I'm glad. She said she thought he was super – and he is. She also said that he made sure that Oxycodone was prescribed for me and hoped I'd get to leave the next day.

July 28, 2012

Yo-yo pain subsiding, the Oxycodone doing its trick. I have always feared narcotics, but my Dad would remind me that, for real pain, narcotics didn't make you loopy or zoned or anything – the meds could attack the pain and give you a plateau of comfort in which to heal. That was true with my C-section, and I stopped taking the drugs around day four, switching to Extra Strength Tylenol.

The Oxycodone was taking enough of an edge off the mastectomy that I could really rest, and engage a bit. I still didn't feel breastless, since I was so heavily bandaged that it felt like a sports bra. My catheter was out and although the IV port still in my wrist, nothing was attached. I was taking meds by mouth and had my leg squeezers off. I had managed to walk a bit today, go to the bathroom, my trusty drains hanging off of my sides like nasty little pineapples. I had been watching with fascination the nurses draining the surgery drains and measuring output. "Yuck", I thought, "that is so alien." Like I was removed from my body and they weren't really attached to me. Dr. Bulldog had been in to visit, checked the expanders and incisions and said that drains normally would come out in a couple of weeks and that he'd do it in his office. "My luck, I'll set the record for having these nasty things," I thought.

Although I hadn't eaten since the Wednesday night before surgery, three days ago, my appetite was only starting to come back, even late into Saturday afternoon. I had eaten the bun off of the top of my chicken sandwich and that was it. Deanna/Helga, who had stayed again last night, had charmed the nurses and they her. She even made her famous potato salad and brought in a big tub of it for our floor this afternoon. Sooooooo, now they would come and check on "us" not just "me." As she prepared her nest for (what I hoped) was our final night, my appetite came back with a vengeance. "Man, I'd like a cheeseburger," I said out loud, knowing full well we had basic snacks, but that the cafeteria had closed hours ago. My favorite team was on duty that night – all men. An older nurse who had retrained when he was laid off of his regular job (mining, I think), a neat nurse about 30, and a young CNA who Deanna had just about adopted. Deanna quietly left the room to "check on something". She brought back something to drink and we talked about our journey during the past three days.

In about 20 minutes, our nurses brought in two sizzling cheeseburgers and some of Deanna's potato salad. Apparently, our resourceful crew had a George Forman in the nurses lounge, along with some hamburger meat and fixings. I almost cried – the humanity, the caring, the over-and-above from these nurses made me feel like everything was going to be fine. (Thanks, guys). I ate most of the burger and some potato salad, as my stomach had shrunk and I didn't want to risk getting an upset stomach. I'm sure the insurance company, who had me slated as out in a day, would cringe if I delayed discharge again due to clandestine burgers. And I missed the Buddy. Bill assured me that he was taking him to tennis, the pool, the playground, keeping his routine as best as they could without "Mommom" there. I wanted to see my boy, to sniff his hair and hear his voice. Tomorrow couldn't come soon enough.

July 29, 2012

Discharge day. With my belly full of burger the night before and the meds doing their thing, I slept better than I had in days – probably weeks since my diagnosis. My discharge was set for the next morning . . . all I needed was the final doctor sign-off, which (miraculously for a hospital) came mid-morning. Buffer pain meds in my bag, as the hospital pharmacy didn't stock Oxycodone to fill, prescription for the same, Deanna had my bags and hers packed and we were headed out the door. The male nurses were off shift by the time I left, so another awesome nurse pushed me down the hall, into the elevator and toward the lobby where my husband and son were waiting outside the glass doors.

I could see David through the window, looking back at me. He broke into the most beautiful, dimpled smile I had ever seen, before or since, and did a little "happy-flap" that he had seen his Mom. I held back my happy tears and told the nurse, "that's my boy" as I tried to raise my hand to wave at him. Mobility-challenges aside, drains securely pinned to the bandage around my chest, I manage to signal the Buddy that I saw him.

The nurse parked my wheelchair beside the van and set the brake, helping me stand. The Buddy watched with fascination and planted a gentle kiss on my lips before bounding into his seat in the van. I thanked the nurse, hugged "Helga" and tried to thank her – no words are adequate to convey all she'd done for me, and allowed my handsome husband to help me into my seat. Awkward and awful – I couldn't swivel well, because I couldn't put my hands down – I couldn't reach the "holy shit" handle to lift myself in, either. When I finally got in, I couldn't reach back to get my seatbelt and dreaded the thought of draping it across my bandaged chest and drains. I held the shoulder part out with my thumb as Bill got it fastened. "You'll break your thumb if we have an accident," he said. One look from me indicated how much I cared about that, so we headed home, all of us sitting in happy silence at our family's reunion.

Grenades and Things I Wish We Had Known

Those damn drains. Bill called them "grenades" because that's exactly what they looked like. Four, clear grenades, sewn into my sides with their tubes disappearing under my skin to parts unknown. I KNEW that I'd have them longer than the average two weeks. I had two of them in for four weeks although the others were removed at around two and a half weeks. I had a revision surgery on my bad side two weeks afterward which necessitated longer drains. On that, apparently, I was still so bruised after the biopsy, that the already-injured tissue wouldn't heal. Even though they were able to save a lot of skin on both sides, they needed to take more from the right side to close the surgery site.

The drains were drained twice every day with Bill monitoring output on a "Drain Log" that he completed. He would take his Drain Log (each drain numbered one through four) to my plastics appointments and be thrilled that they would want copies for my file. Bill would also note the color of the drainage and whether there was any odor to monitor for infection. Gross.

DRAIN LOG

date/time	#1	#2	#3	#4	comments

One of my remaining drains also was clogged and, when cleared, flowed like crazy for a few days, which also prevented its removal. Bill went to all the appointments and was fascinated, watching the tube snake out from under my skin when the stitches were removed and drains pulled.

Among the annoyances of the drains is that there was nowhere to put them. So they didn't hang and pull at my skin (I was assured there was no danger) Bill kept a bandage around my chest with an ace bandage on top of that and the drains safety pinned to the ace. We'd pin them to the top of my pants when changing bandages. My husband will never work in munitions . . . he dropped one of my drains once and I gagged and almost passed out. I slept largely reclined for the first couple of weeks, just because it was much more comfortable with the drains. The tops of the drains have little holes to clip to the bandages and it is sooooo much more comfortable to clip them to the front instead of the side.

The worst part was trying to go about my life . . . with drains. Getting in and out of the car, trying to sleep, but not being able to get my arms next to my sides, nothing to really wear . . . . As part of helping David transition into his new classrooms each year (transitioning is tough for many Aspies) we always go to the school the day before he starts. His awesome elementary school and teachers have it together for him to see his room, his desk and his locker. The teacher also lets him know what is expected first thing in the morning, where to stick his lunch, where to return homework, etc. so he can start with a clear vision for himself. Transition works wonders – for almost everything. I had never missed the day-before transition and wasn't about to for his fourth grade – drains or no drains. I wore a stretch top with a wrap over it and stood to the side, afraid of getting bumped, watching my pride-and-joy figure out his new surroundings. David left the transition ready to conquer school the next day. Lord-willing, I won't miss any other transitions either.

Drains aside, a big key to recovery was button-up shirts - BIG roomy button-up shirts - I wore Bill's XXL silk Hawaiian shirts for the first week, both for coverage and ease of getting in and out with some of the arm-mobility issues in the early days. I'd put my bad side with the lymph removal in first and then slide the other arm in as it has better mobility.

Once home, I'd wiggle my fingers, raise arms, bend elbows, etc. as far as I could – as I'd had simple mastectomy on my left side and modified radical (sampled some nodes) on the right side, the chest muscles aren't touched, so, other than discomfort and stretching (not really painful), moving will help prevent lymphedema which IS painful and can become chronic.

Pain medication also has the tendency to make you itchy. When I was in the hospital, I would beg whomever was handy to scratch my back (gently, as the nerves were cross-wired back there, too), until they couldn't anymore. Helga came up with the great idea to use the tritons that hold cards in flower bouquets for the job. Man, did they work great. Unfortunately, when I had enough mobility to use them myself, I was constantly over-zealous and broke many little tritons, scratching and scratching, the itch that wouldn't quit. Note to self . . . the clear ones truly disappear on the carpet and hurt when you step on them – sorry, Honey.

My hair was so funky after four days of not washing it that I could barely stand myself. Unfortunately, I couldn't get the incisions wet for a few weeks. My brilliant husband again saved the day. I stood in the shower, naked other than the bandages and damn drains, inside a massive trashbag opened like a skirt at the bottom and with the tie part tied around my neck over a neck-towel and under the trash bag tie to catch leaks. That let him wash my hair and legs and backside without getting the dressings wet. We'd turn on the shower, I'd step in (holding the trash bag ties tightly), get my hair wet, and we'd turn it off. He'd lather, turn it on, I'd step in and rinse and he'd turn it off. He'd use water running from the bath faucet to wash and rinse my body in a sort of "sponge bath", but it felt so good to be clean.

Finally, the constipation . . . I know, just when I can't get any sexier with no breasts, drain-grenades, funky hair and men's Hawaiian shirts. I seriously don't understand how people can get hooked on narcotics. Besides the sleeping and itching, no one told me how they constipate you after more than a few days. Getting up and down from the toilet without touching anything (drains) is difficult, but I was camped there for two days – miserable at not being able to go. That was the worst of my "at home" pain. Finally, after much begging by Bill, I had an at-home enema . . . he took the Buddy downstairs, I was screaming so much as it took effect. The doctor prescribed Sennekot-S for the evenings and to dissolve and drink Miralax though the day afterward. Let's not go into how challenging lack of arm mobility makes getting clean "back there" . . . suffice it to say, it's the only time I wished to be French . . . Bidet, anyone?

I wish they would have told me about constipation from pain medication before I got to that point. Drains aside, that was the worst. I also wonder how anyone could be addicted to pain medication . . . constipation, dizziness and itchy skin isn't my idea of a good buzz.

August 13, 2012

Heading to Plastics for a post-surgery follow up. As Bill and I walk back through the doors of the same practice suite post-surgery that I did beforehand, I am chagrined at my previous opinion of plastic surgeons catering to vanity and am thankful to have the option. The Buddy is with our Godsend, Sarah, as she continues to watch him this summer like in the past. I remain grateful, too, that we chose to have the surgery and reconstruction in the city where we live. I have friends and wives of friends who are driving to Duke or Johns Hopkins for appointments and follow-ups when we have the national standard of care available right here. I can't imagine driving four hours for a drain check. Stamina-wise, I get fatigued so easily just walking to the car and sitting, trying to position the seat-belt so it doesn't tug or push on the damn drains. I'm irrationally afraid of the airbag . . . I've never been in an accident where one was deployed, but my sliced and diced chest and dangling grenades make me feel certain that it's going to let loose and cause grave bodily harm . . . just on my side.

My sweet husband parks as close as he can. He's afraid to drop me off in front, I'm so unsteady on my feet. I've been off the pain meds for a few days, but am still dizzy and tired as my body gets used to its missing parts and shifting blood-flow. Getting in and out of the van is getting easier, but I didn't realize how much I use my hands to swivel and slide in the car – forget pulling it closed, I can't do it just yet. Bill comes around to get me, carries my purse and patiently lets me shuffle my way to the door, into the building and up the elevator.

It's the first time I've been here that I've <u>felt</u> like a patient. The other times, I was whole – now I'm broken. I sign in and sit down. No one in the waiting room is particularly interested in me. Maybe I don't look as broken as I feel. Maybe they are broken, too. In fairly short order, Bill and I are called back to the room. Vitals are taken, now-routine questions are asked by the kind nurse and I'm given the gown to put on "open to the front." Bill helps me put it on and gently slips my arms in the holes. Thank God the gown is over-sized – so helpful to not struggle into it.

In a few minutes, Dr. Bulldog knocks and steps into the room. This is the first time Bill has met him, but they hit it off immediately. My husband never meets a stranger and Dr. Bulldog always has a smile. Bill proudly hands over the drain report from the past couple of weeks and puffs up even more when the nurse wants a copy. They gently unclip the drains from the ace bandage I still wear over the gauze wrappings and reclip them to the top of the yoga pants I'm wearing. Slowly, slowly, the doctor unwinds the bandage and removes the gauze.

I still can't look down and keep my eyes on my husband. Dr. Bulldog seems pleased with the left side (the non-offending, never cancerous, "good side") and says that I'm healing well. As for my "bad side", he says "I really don't like the look of this part of the incision" as he points to an area I won't look at and can't feel. Bill leans in and nods, keeping the smile on his face for my benefit. My old paramedic is fazed by nothing and knows I look to his reaction for guidance on whether to worry or not. "Why do you think that is?" Bill asks. Dr. Bulldog said that the area was where the biopsy was and was still bruised by the time of surgery. Part of the incision went through already bruised tissue, which has a tough time healing. "Makes sense," Bill said.

"What does that mean?" I asked. "Can we just see if it will heal on its own? Or what can we do?" Dr. Bulldog smiles and pats my hand – not patronizingly, but reassuringly – fine line, but he walks it brilliantly. "We can do a revision surgery, just on that side. I'll just take a little more skin in that area and eliminate the bruised area and the incision should heal well. It's nothing compared to what you've already been through and should be an out-patient procedure."

I looked at Bill and, with that look of confidence that gets me through, he nodded and said, "when can we get it done? Bethie has her first Oncology this Friday and we don't know how to prepare for that." The nurse slid out to check his surgery schedule while Bill and Dr. Bulldog talked about what I could expect during the revision. Admittedly, I was only half-listening – my mind kept saying "another surgery . . . I'll never be through this." The nurse popped back in and said that he had an opening that Thursday, the 14th, and would that work. "Absolutely," Bill and I both agreed. The only way out of this nightmare is through.

Heavy Healing

Aside from the things I wish I knew after surgery, I marvel at the strangeness of how the body compensates for trauma. Although I hated the pain medication side effects, they did put me to sleep and I slept soundly and pain-free for hours at a time. My blessed son understood "surgery" (but still doesn't know "cancer") and would generally be there when I awoke. Although the Buddy is truly all boy, and was nine at the time, I'd awaken to find a scattering of his favorite toys around the bed, where he'd quietly played while I slept. Or he'd sit next to me in the chair beside the bed, playing handheld games and jump up to bring something for me.

I'll never know how much seeing me like that hurt his kid psyche, or if it did. I do know my son says the word "surgery" with a worried reverence, even now. And, out of the blue, he asked me seven or eight months later if I was done with my surgery. I reassured him that I was (Lord-willing). He then asked, "may I sit on your lap again?" With my heart both full and breaking, I gathered my tall, nearly 10 year-old on my lap, hugging and rocking him, realizing how much I had missed it, too.

Every time I would get out of the bed in the guestroom, I would stand straight and my body would do an almost-convulsive stretch, as if I hadn't move any muscles while I was prone. Stopping the stretch was impossible, the mechanism wired into my healing. I slept in the guestroom for months, afraid of being poked in the chest or drains at first, feeling so lousy with therapies that I was afraid I'd awaken vomiting, and my lifelong insomnia was now compounded by fear of never getting the things done in life that I needed to do for my younger son and my family. Despite sleeping in separate beds for the only time in our marriage, these months of getting through tough treatments were the most-connected that we had ever been.

Another issue I had with healing was that I was constantly chilled, as if my body couldn't regulate its thermostat after my amputations. The fun part (tongue in cheek) was when the involuntary stretch would coincide with the wave of chills. And if you are wondering if you get phantom nipple-erections after a mastectomy – you do. At least I did. The first time was a little shocking. You hear about phantom pains with missing limbs . . . so it struck me as the chill took hold that it may be the case for mastectomies. I waited and, either my mind took over or the nerves remembered what used to be, but, there it was . . . or there they were. The sensation of nipple-erections without nipples. I would have sworn they were still there. I would have checked, but that entails looking down. Don't look down – can't look back.

August 16, 2012

"Here we go," I thought, moving quietly down the stairs in the pre-dawn, so to not awaken my sleeping son. I was up well before the alarm sounded. Bill was already downstairs, ready to take me to the hospital for revision surgery. Sarah would be here soon, to be here when my son awoke. "God bless, Sarah", I said for the millionth time since she came into our lives a few years back and for the thousandth time in the past few weeks. She's uncommonly kind and responsible for any person, much less an adult in her late teens.

Bill got up from the kitchen table and gave me a hug, gently so as to not pull my remaining drains. During my post-surgery check-up, Dr. Bulldog had removed the two on my left side. He showed Bill where to watch on my chest wall and, as he snipped the stiches and gently pulled, Bill could see the drain tubes snake silently from under my skin and out of my body. There is no pain, just a gentle tugging like stitches being removed. Gross.

"Why am I hungrier on mornings that I can't eat than I am on the mornings I can?" I asked, rhetorically. "It's the coffee I miss the most." That *is* true – I'm a 3-cups-before 10:00 person, down significantly from my days waiting tables.

"When is Sarah coming?" Bill asked, although he knew already. "At 7:00," I answered, as we lapsed into silence, each comforted being with the other, but isolated in our own thoughts. As the morning of surgery means no hair products, make-up or jewelry, I had little to distract me while waiting. I had slipped into another of Bill's Hawaiian shirts this morning – although mobility *is getting better and better, I'm still sore and the drains still bulky on my right side. So I checked the refrigerator again, making sure the Buddy had his favorites stocked – not just for today, but for a few days while I recovered. Extra favorites for Sarah were tucked away as well. I laid out some clothes for David for today for him to pick from and blankets in front of the TV for him to nest in when he came downstairs. It was hot (again) and Sarah was still on crutches. This entailed her own surgery, plates and screws, so I'm sure she was relieved that it was too miserable to go outside, much.*

At a few minutes before 7:00, Sarah pulled into the driveway. We had parked the van at on the street the night before, so she had a shorter distance to navigate in. Ever-present smile on her pretty face, Sarah crutched inside, set down her bag and threw Bill and me out the door. "We'll be fine," she said, "text me if you need anything." And with that, she closed the door, locking it behind her.

My sweet husband, walking on my "good side" held my arm as we moved down the driveway in the early morning light, helped me into the van and closed the door (hate that motion). We road through our quiet neighborhood on our way to the hospital, General Division, not Memorial, for the out-patient procedure. "Did you pre-register?" Bill asked, knowing full well that I did. "Yes," I answered, "I should just be able to check in at the window."

When we got to the hospital, he dropped me off at the front door, so I didn't need to expend my precious and scant energy getting from the parking garage. "First time in this hospital since Dad was discharged after his surgery," I thought. "Could it only have been two and a half months ago? Feels like a lifetime." I walked up to the empty bank of windows and was warmly greeted by the Intake representative. Giving my name, she briskly pulled my packet, asked my name and date of birth . . . and of course asked, "and how would you like to handle your deductible today?" We're blessed with great healthcare and am constantly grateful and guilty knowing that others aren't so blessed.

By the time I wrote the check and was banded, Bill had joined me. We walked down the ramp to Day Surgery, him carrying books and snacks, me carrying the lump in my throat. At the bottom of the ramp, we took a left at the bank of elevators and up to the Surgery window. The same professional, but pleasant, gentleman who was there when Dad had his surgery on June 1st, was there today. It was somehow comforting to see his familiar face. He told Bill to wait in the waiting room while they gowned me up, started my IV and the rest of the surgery prep. "I need him to help me get into the gown," I said, not mentioning that I needed him for reassurance, as well. "The nurse will help you," he replied, kindly, seeing through my ruse, "they'll call him back as soon as they can."

I was led into one of the curtained stalls and indeed helped into a gown – my nurse was non-plussed to see my mid-section bound like a mummy and drains hanging from my right side. She asked the standard questions, "What is your procedure?" "Can you mark the side of your procedure?" "I see latex allergy . . . what does it do to you?" and brought a warm blanket for my lap. Love those!

Shortly thereafter she started the IV in my left arm, putting a pink "limb restricted" band on my right. Some doctors say it will be at least seven or 10 years before I can have blood drawn or a blood pressure cuff on the right side – the risk of post-lymph removal lymphedema remains high for years after surgery. Some doctors say "never" – I was grateful that the nurse thought of the band before I had to ask. Then Bill was brought back to sit with me. We barely had 10 minutes together before the orderly arrived to take me. "I love you," I said, "see you soon." Bill kissed me and smiled, but the smile didn't reach his worried eyes. The orderly drove my bed around the tight corners better than I drive my poor, beat-up van. We made small-talk during the trip, but I didn't process a word. He parked me against the wall in the middle of the staging room, locked the wheels on my bed, patted my foot and said "good luck" before hustling away on another run.

I tried not to look at the other surgery patients being wheeled in – overwhelmed with my own misery, I couldn't bear to see it in the eyes of another. "How is this me? How is this nightmare my reality?" I thought, as tears rolled down the sides of my face and into my hair on the pillow. The nurses, physicians assistants, nursing assistants, lab workers bustled around the small room, fully gowned and wearing their "lunch lady" hats. One pretty nurse was showing her manicure to another . . . "Look – I did blue and gold with little 'WVs" for the football game this weekend." "Cute!" her friend exclaimed, while they planned their weekend wardrobes. They weren't being insensitive, but I had to suppress the urge to scream at them . . . . talking about manicures and football outfits. I'm freaking out about cancer, surgery, recovery, my boys, my life and they go on living their lives . . . how DARE they.

Pulling me from the brink of an ugly meltdown, a slight woman with a serious face and great smile, slid silently up to the side of my bed. "Hi," she said "I'm the nurse anesthetist who will be assisting the Anesthesiologist during your surgery today. When was the last time you had anything to eat? Would you please open your mouth so I can look at your airway? Any dentures or partials? Any prior problems with anesthesia?" As with the first round of anesthesia three weeks prior, I answered, opened my mouth, shook my head as she noted my responses. "The Anesthesiologist will be here shortly. Who is your surgeon?" she asked. "Dr. Bulldog," I responded. "I had breast cancer and a double mastectomy a few weeks ago. I need revision surgery on one side." I don't know why I feel the need to lay it out in full, every time, but I do. Is it to justify why I'm seeing a plastic surgeon? Is it because saying it enough might take the horror of my reality away? Or is it because I still can't believe it?

My rambling didn't phase her one bit. "My sister had breast cancer," she said, without further detail. "You'll be fine. And we all love Dr. Bulldog – he's a very good surgeon and treats everyone like a part of his team. We're just waiting for him to get here to start. <u>Your</u> surgeon is usually right on time," she laughed conspiratorially. She smiled again, hung my chart on the end of my bed and walked into the back room.

A few minutes later (and a few minutes early for my procedure) Dr. Bulldog entered the room, coffee in hand. He didn't linger at the chart area or desk and came right up to me with a "Hi, Beth – are you ready to get started?" Immediately, I felt human again – I felt "seen". Didn't call me "Mrs. Minear", didn't check my chart, didn't catch up with his work peeps (who ALL stood straighter when he entered the room) – he looked me in the eye, called me by my name, held my hand and made it <u>bearable</u> – doable. "It won't be anything like last time," he promised. "You should be home by mid-afternoon, sore, but not nearly in as much pain." I nodded, trying not to cry again, this time in relief and gratitude. Dr. Bulldog gave my hand a final squeeze before I was rolled into surgery.

In surgery, my anesthesiologist came in, gowned and ready to go. "When was the last time you had anything to eat? Would you please open your mouth so I can look at your airway? Any dentures or partials? Any prior problems with anesthesia?" I found myself thinking that they must all have a script . . . and that airline flight attendants with their rote speeches had something to aspire to. The surgery became busier and busier, with more disciplines joining my party. I cautioned them about my drains and mobility on the right side as a mask was laid over my nose and mouth. A few breaths and that was it.

August 24, 2012

Sweet son off to school and Bill and I are heading to my oncology appointment. Making it to the originally-scheduled appointment last Friday didn't work. Revision surgery the day before wiped me out. When Bill called to reschedule, they urged him to get me in as soon as possible. "Is that a sign?" I wondered, "was my cancer so advanced that more body parts need to be removed?" I tried to put it out of my mind. No one had called to say whether any of my lymph nodes were engaged so I guess we'd find out today.

I prayed silently, "Lord, please guide our treatment decisions today, if decisions are to be made for further treatment. We trust in your guidance and wisdom and will hear you when you speak to us." I've always prayed in my head throughout my life – for as long as I can remember. Sometimes only a "Thank you, Lord" for a small gift of grace, or a "Please let the Buddy have a smooth day today", which is my significant prayer every morning for David. Praise and prayer – although admittedly I ask more than I thank – not for things, but for grace in situations. Our pastor says that he believes that God speaks to us now as in Biblical days – we're just so full of static in our lives, we just don't listen or chalk it up to coincidence. I have always believed that God gives us messages – and I have tried to follow what I am given. So today I head to oncology in full belief that, if a decision is to be made, God will give direction.

For Dad's cancer treatment, he was taken on by Dr. Lifeline, a nationally-renowned oncologist who has practiced for decades, but who sparingly takes new patients. He took on Dad's treatment since they had known each other for decades. He accepted me as a patient because of Dad. Dr. Gyne tried to not let me get my hopes up when we were discussing oncologist consultation options. "I'm going to see Dr. Lifeline," I told him. "That whole practice group is good. May I suggest Dr. Other - it's unlikely you'll get Dr. Lifeline as he doesn't typically take new patients," he said. I smiled despite my anxiety this morning, as I eased myself into the car, remembering the conversation.

Bill and I drove the short distance from home to Dr. Lifeline's office. The Oncology group is in the same building as Dr. Healer, my surgeon, and right across from the hospital where I had my mastectomy. I try not to look at the hospital, as we pull up and Bill drops me off in the front – the memories of post-surgery pain still to fresh. My stamina is still awful, although I'm working on it, so I sit out front until he joins me. We walk through the foyer of the building to the rear of the first floor, where the oncology group has its practice, sharing space with its infusion services. Opening the door, I'm struck by two thoughts . . . first, that there are so many patients sitting in the crowded waiting room, and, second, that the waiting room isn't as scary or ominous as I feared.

I walked to the window to sign in and was greeted with warm smiles without a trace of pity. Giving my name, I received some documents and was asked if I'd participate in a "Distress Study" being conducted. Purely voluntary, but I agreed, wanting to see if I could plot my level of distress on paper. On advice of Friday in Dr. Healer's office, a few days before, Bill had picked up the thick packet of forms to fill out for my intake into oncology. It took about 40 minutes to fill out at home. I was grateful to be able to hand it over this morning, skipping that step in the waiting room so I could focus on calming my nerves. I sat down with the "Distress Scale" and scanned through the questions. I rated my distress on the paper thermometer, and then went through the different questions as to whether I had problems with childcare, insurance, financial, family, etc.. "No, no, no . . ." I answered for most of the questions. My relative blessings shown to me, I went back to the thermometer and revised my distress downward.

As I was finishing, the door opened next to the intake window. "Minear", I was called. Taking the clipboard with me, Bill and I went back with the nurse, handing it to him when we reached the side room. "Just getting some vitals and bloodwork," he said, "then we'll send you back to the waiting room, unless an exam room becomes available." I climb on the scale and am amazed that I've lost 20 pounds in five weeks. Eight of it was boob, but still . . . 20 pounds? The nurse drew blood and checked the rest of my vitals. Bill helped me out of the black wrap that I had been wearing lately, as it provided a great deal of camouflage for my new shape, especially as I was still carrying the last, damn drain. He and I were largely silent, polite to the nurse, but lost together and separately in our thoughts for the pending examination. Sticking his head out of the room and peering to the right, the nurse said, "we have a room for you. Follow me, please."

Bill draped the black wrap loosely over my shoulders and followed me down the hall. "Disrobe from the waist up and put the gown on open to the back, if you would," I was told, as we were ushered into a large, normal-looking exam room. The door closed and Bill again helped me undress and gown up. Mobility limitations are exhausting.

We waited for probably 20 minutes before the knock on the door. Opening slightly, around the corner peered what had to be the good doctor. I immediately felt at ease. Dr. Lifeline is a slight man, with kind, bright eyes and perpetual smile. He sported a traditional white lab coat, set off by a really funky, indescribable tie. None of that gave me the ease I felt. Maybe it was how I'd built him up in my mind or the hushed awe I had been hearing from friends when they found out who my Oncologist is, or something explainable psychologically. Whatever it is (and it sounds strange even to me), Dr. Lifeline has an energy that . . . well . . . glows. "I'll be in here shortly," he said, "could I get you coffee or something to drink, something to eat?" We assured him that we were fine and he retreated from view.

About 10 minutes later, the doctor knocked again and came in. He shook hands with both Bill and me, and asked me to get on the exam table. I mentioned that I was still wrapped with the ace bandage and gauze from last week's revision surgery, as well as still having a drain. Dr. Lifeline peeked at the bandages and said, "Well, I won't disturb any of that this time. We'll do the rest of the exam." The good doctor proceeded to give me the best physical examination I can ever remember having. He palpitated across my torso, listening with a practiced ear. He firmly examined the nodes in my neck, arm pits (gently under my right arm) and groin, took pulses in my feet, checked reflexes and measured bilateral strength with my arms, hands and legs. I examined his face for any signs of concern or horror, but Dr. Lifeline, kept the same pleasant expression on his face, although you could see him "filing" his results in his head.

"You can get dressed and then we'll talk" he said. A few minutes later, having given us time to get me redressed, Dr. Lifeline knocked and returned, perching on a stool at the corner of the countertop, pulling many sheets of blank paper before him as he did so. He started reading my pathology report, jotting notes and talking outloud as he did . . . "Right modified radical mastectomy, left simple mastectomy . . . nothing "simple" about it is there . . . some nodal engagement . . . "I caught my breath and looked at Bill. Dr. Lifeline looked at us, "you hadn't had the pathology results?" he asked. I shook my head, unable to speak. Where before I was afraid, now I was terrified. Although waiting the nine short days between diagnosis and surgery, I thought I felt evil creeping under my right armpit, I had kept it to myself. Likely in my mind, but maybe it was my body telling me in advance. Bill had been convinced that there would be no nodes – I felt in my heart otherwise.

Dr. Lifeline said simply, "it'll be all right. We'll talk after we get treatment planned." Writing longhand, for eight full pages, he went through talking out loud, telling us, teaching us as he wrote. "Let's see . . . Mammogram July 5, OB-GYN appointment July 6, Biopsy July 12, Diagnosis July 17, Surgery July 26 . . . wow, that's good," he remarked. "She has had good care, so far," Bill said, "each of them kept planning ahead." Dr. Lifeline replied, "that's how it supposed to go . . . should go, but it doesn't always." He looked down and kept writing, and talking, walking through the standard chemotherapy protocol and radiation protocol of 30 rounds of radiation, followed by 5 years of Tamoxifen, another 5 years of Arimedex. "In going through all of this, and I'm recommending it all, we'll reduce chance of recurrence by 45 % and mortality by 35%. Do you want me to calculate your risks?" He looked up expectantly. Bill and I looked at each other in shock and horror . . . not at the kind doctor, but just the thought. Dr. Lifeline read the looks and said "never mind . . . not necessary" and put down his pen.

He turned to me and said, "I'd like you to consider one of the drug trials that you may be a candidate for." My mind immediately went to **"terminal – nothing but trials will really work"**, but I kept my face blank and let him continue. There is one in it's third clinical test . . . 1800 women nationwide are going to be in this final test. We have 10 of those 1800 slots here. We'll need to make sure that there are no metastases anywhere else (which I don't anticipate) and screen you for any other issues, like heart output. I see where you already had a CT Scan, which showed no mets, so that's a great start. Now, if you want the standard chemotherapy protocol, that's your choice. If you choose to be in the clinical trial, there is a 50-50 chance that you'll be randomized into the group that gets the standard anyway . . . there is no guarantee you'll get the proposed course."

My sweet husband, being more medically-inclined than I, asked, "what is different about the trial course of action? What are they trying to confirm?" I'm glad he asked . . . I'm still so overwhelmed by everything, I'm not thinking well. Dr. Lifeline replied, "the standard chemotherapy for this is so heart-toxic. I really don't want to see your wife come in here in 10 or 15 years in heart failure, with swollen ankles, unable to breathe. We're trying to mitigate the heart-toxic drug by and giving a different regimen, and the third round of trials is to prove it's just as good as the standard." And with that sentence came a wave of hope – it *didn't blot out the blanket of despair, but did roll it down to let me peek out a bit.*

Beyond the faith I have that God is always in control and knows what He is doing, I now had the "earthly" hope of avoiding effects "10 to 15 years" in the future. "Before you decide, if you are interested in hearing more, I'd like you to meet my colleague with the National Cancer Institute. Her office is upstairs, but I'll call her down if you are interested." Bill and I nodded simultaneously, without even looking at each other. Dr. Lifeline's ever-present, genuine smile grew even bigger, "great" he said, and dashed out of the room.

Bill and I sat in silence. A few minutes later, the good doctor came back, bringing with him a beautiful nurse, who (I swear) matches his glow. "This is Karen", he introduced. "She doesn't work for the hospital or for me, but is with the National Cancer Institute helping us to get into trials, monitor treatment and results and acting as patient advocate. If you decide to do the trial, whether you get the standardized treatment or the new protocol, along with the other oversight this office gives to all of our patients, you also get Karen and monitoring for life, even beyond when treatment with me would normally end. I'll let you all talk and will check back later." And with that, he dashed out of the room again.

Karen sat down on the stool vacated by Dr. Lifeline only a few minutes ago. Smiling, she spoke "he's so good. Honestly, you are getting the best care. He's brilliant and such a kind, kind man. I work with so many oncologists in the area, not just at CAMC, and I learn so much from Dr. Lifeline. I've told him that he can't ever retire – if I get sick, he's going to need to be on my team for treatment decisions." Being the daughter of a doctor, my Dad had always said that if you want the real skinny on doctors, ask the nurses who they'd go to if they needed a doctor. Her few words to break the ice spoke to my fears.

Moving cleanly to the diagnosis and treatment discussion, Karen said, "whatever you decide needs to be right for you. You know you have an excellent prognosis. Your cancer was double-positive. That means it was hormone-fed, and is hormone-receptive to treatment." My mind and my heart struggled to take it in – "excellent prognosis? Really?" I was confused, too, at the "your cancer" part . . . "Isn't breast cancer, breast cancer? There are different kinds?" I thought. I hadn't Googled anything to self-diagnose, to freak myself out or come in thinking I knew it all. I asked Bill to not, either. We wanted to come in with open minds and a clean slate – not to be uninformed, but preventing being "ill-informed." I still haven't. I have flesh and blood doctors, not Google-graduates.

Talking to Karen for the first time, I said, "I want to do my part for moving ahead treatment for women. I know that my treatment was developed from the treatment of thousands of women before me who paved the way for the rest of us. I can't risk it, though, if they already know that the trial isn't as good as the standard chemotherapy, heart-toxic or not." Going on, I explained myself by revealing what I don't typically in a first conversation without the Buddy with me. "I have a son who has Asperger's, on the Autism Spectrum. I need to out-live my son, even if only for a day." Karen reached over to me and grasped my hand in understanding, her beautiful, serene eyes shining with tears. "My daughter has Autism. I know how that feels and know what you are thinking.

This protocol is in the third trial. There are no guarantees, even in the standard therapies, but if it performs like expected, it will become a new standard." And with her revelation of her daughter's Autism, the connection was made. We special needs' Mommas connect immediately, in general, but Karen's disclosure was the sign that I asked God for this morning . . . "If there is a treatment choice to be made, Lord, please show me the way." He did.

"I'd like to be included in the trial," I said, a little breathlessly. I looked over to Bill. Without releasing my hand Karen reached her other hand over to his. "Bill?" she asked. My big, kind husband broke down, "I just can't lose my wife" he sobbed, "whatever gives her the best chance to stay with me as long as she can, I'm in for." Karen let go of both of us and grabbed tissues for all of us. "I think this trial is a good choice for the long term" she confirmed her belief. "There is no guarantee you'll get the new protocol . . . it's randomized at NCI and you are only identified by a number. I'll know you're number here, but have no way of knowing how the computer will place you. Let me get Dr. Lifeline and we'll plan." She reached out and gave me another hand-squeeze and stepped out.

A few minutes later, both Karen and Dr. Lifeline returned together. "So, you're interested in the trial," he said, "good, good. We have a few tests we need you to have done before we can submit your name. You had the CT Scan already, but we'll need a bone scan to rule out metastesis there, too. I don't expect to find anything, but you won't be considered if there is metastesis. We will also need to get a thyroid ultrasound and a heart refraction to test your cardiac output. Regardless of whether you do the trial or not, you will likely want to get an infusion port for the *chemotherapy – it'll save your veins. Dr. Healer is a whiz – he can probably insert one for you in his sleep."*

"More tests, more worry," I thought. You'd think I'd welcome confirmation of the doctor's belief that we wouldn't find anything else, but all I could think of is that they've made a mistake on the CT Scan and the next tests will show cancer everywhere. Still, even finding more gives me shot at comprehensive treatment. Karen's calm voice pierced my thoughts, "I'll get the appointments set up in the next week, including the port installation. You call me after each appointment and let me know how it went and I'll keep inputting the results. Since we only have 10 slots, I want you to get one of them." I nodded. Dr. Lifeline resumed writing for the next few minutes. He had copies made for me of what he had written and Bill and I left him and Karen shortly thereafter, leaving the surreal World of Oncology to pick up the Buddy from school.

Planning and Preparation

While I have always been a "Type A" over-achiever . . . a "put my head down and plow through" the tough tasks kind of person . . . I had never been a planner before having David. When I was really young, my mother likes to tell how unprepared for school I was every morning, physically, not mentally. My little sister would turn out with hair done, clothes together, matching this-and-that, while I struggled out of the house, hair in a wet pony-tail and pulling on shoes as I'd go. When going to a week-long camp as a teenager, mother would worry out loud as she surveyed my open, but still empty trunk the night before we left. My sister would have been packed for a week. Even traveling overseas as an adult in my late twenties, I rarely had hotel rooms booked across multiple country treks, preferring instead to see where I was at the end of the day and figuring it out from there.

Law school changed that a bit. I had three jobs as I went through my third year, so being prepared was the only way to succeed. Having the Buddy made me into a planner and a preparer. As "high functioning" as he is with Asperger's (whatever that means), he still has issues with change of routine and disorganization. My Plan Bs have Plan Bs (and Plan Cs many times). It has worked well – for us and him. I can count maybe a dozen times in his first decade that I hadn't thought through all of the possible outcomes of a trip, event or scenario (or had and one surprised me) and there was a resulting incident. Otherwise, David has gone everywhere and done everything we have without much issue – tons of planning and packing on the front end, but nothing on the back end.

How do you prepare for chemotherapy? Almost five months of it given in three week rounds? My freezer isn't big enough even if I had felt like cooking and freezing for a week with limited mobility and strength. I had about 10 days before my first round, and had tests, appointments and a port to be installed under my skin in addition to prepping for after chemotherapy. So I did what any Type-A mother would do – I cleaned out my linen closet. I controlled what I could, leaving the scary thoughts in the background of meaningless focus and made myself busy with nothing.

The Buddy had been in school for a couple of weeks and doing fine in the clothes department. It was still scorching hot, so his shorts were perfect. While helping to care for Dad, working through the Derecho, my diagnosis, surgery, etc., I had not planned for Fall and Winter clothes for David like I usually did in years past. He's easy to shop for as far as Asperger's goes. As long as clothes aren't too tight in the neck or waist, have no tags, socks have seams at the end of the foot, not over the toe . . . he does fine. The first thing I did in leading up to therapy was order clothes to get the Buddy through to February. We had a massive try-on party in his bedroom one afternoon (he hates it, but was so patient). Bill and I boxed everything that didn't fit to send to a family friend's son who is 18 months younger and then figured out what gaps David had in his Fall/Winter wardrobe that I would need to order.

My next order of business was to take care of Christmas shopping – hard to think about in August, but I knew that I'd be immuno-suppressed for the next few months, so I wouldn't be able to shop in person. I do the majority on line now anyway, as I dislike crowds and stores are less shopper-friendly than I remember 20 years ago. Still . . . getting it all done, on-line in a few days was challenging. With the get-well cards that kept coming (and still do), I got into routine to send "thank yous" for each one a few at a time until I had thanked every one. I planned to do the same with gifts as they came in – wrap a few at a time and put them aside, forgiving myself for the two piles that remained in the guest bedroom (to-be-wrapped and wrapped).

Finally, cleaning and laundry. With my schedule at work and with appointments, I couldn't do to the extent that I wanted . . . the top to bottom and leaving nothing out. I did thin out my own closet, Bill washed everything and we put away and we rearranged the linen closet and kitchen cabinets. Don't ask me why (and Bill didn't as we did them) . . . it benefitted us not at all throughout, but I HAD to get it done before starting chemotherapy. Mostly to get my mind off of what was to come. I had no actual idea of what to expect aside from the horror stories of the torture that I was to endure. Like stories of childbirth that leave no one ever wanting to have children – ever – I had never heard a "piece of cake" chemotherapy story. Even the word is always shortened to "chemo" instead of addressing what it is . . . "therapy."

Since I had no way to know what to expect, I wiped expectations from my mind and instead planned and prepared for what no one can prepare adequately for.

Drug Trial Gauntlet

Getting into drug trials for me had three distinct parts: 1) having the fortitude, planning and insistence to get them done in a week; 2) getting the results needed to qualify; and 3) grace of God blessing the process. Although I struggled with worrying that I would somehow compromise my care and, therefore, my prognosis by agreeing to this trial, I know that there are no guarantees no matter what course. I believe that God clearly showed the path I was meant to take so I gave over my worries to Him. I also know of women who made it through standard chemotherapy and have died of heart-attacks at a relatively-young age from the ravages it can wreak.

To be a candidate for the trial (with no guarantee that I will be randomized into the new regimen), I needed to be free of metastasis anywhere else. I had already had x-rays and the CT scan pre-surgery, but needed a bone scan as well. The final drain came out on Monday, August 27, 2012, making it much easier to maneuver and position onto the scanner. I also had a thyroid ultrasound to make sure it was functioning well (and found nodules – more about that later). Finally, I needed an echocardiogram to measure my heart refraction to make sure it was adequate for the task. After each test or each appointment, Karen Shirey, who by now I was already thinking of as "Karen Angel", would push the offices to get me in and would pull the test results and let me know that I was still a candidate.

When the final result was in, my name was turned into a number and randomized with the National Cancer Institute for this drug trial. At that point, although the waiting game was nearing the end, I felt both anxiety and peace. I believed that God had led me to participate in the trial and that I would be in the new drug group to potentially protect my heart from the ravages of standard chemotherapy. But since God's directions aren't always spelled out, I also could have been directed by Him to serve as a member of the control group with standard therapy to advance science for others. I was anxious to be in the drug trial group, but peaceful in whatever was chosen for me.

The day after my heart echo, the last test, we had the results – I had been randomized into the drug trial group. Bill said that he knew that would be where I would land. I was less sure of the landing, but grateful that's how it ended. Although Karen warned me that the course would be tough, minimizing the heart toxic effects of standard therapy was a good thing. I was ready for the challenge.

Chemotherapy – Observations of a Foggy Mind

Just the abbreviation "CHEMO" is enough to shake the bravest of brave. Through everything I had been through to this point, the concept of chemotherapy was one on which I'd had an odd relationship. I naively had thought (pre-cancer) that, "to be on the safe side", maybe folks should elect to have a round of chemotherapy at different points in their lives to kill of wayward cancer cells. I didn't realize that there were different therapies for different types of cancer (breast, lung, colon, etc.) and different cancers within each type of cancer (i.e. triple-negative, double positive, etc. for breast cancer) . . . or even different options for chemotherapy for a single diagnosis.

When I was diagnosed . . . before knowing that I had some nodal engagement, knowing what type of cancer that I had and even before the biopsy came back as positive . . . I both wanted and feared chemotherapy. The fear part is a normal, rational response to that which evoked images of tortured souls, gaunt and bedridden, wretching into basins while they waste away. The "want" part is a little strange, I gather. I've spoken to more than a few who have gone through chemotherapy and other fellow breast cancer Survivors who did not need it. Although a few have said they understood what I was saying, I haven't had anyone agree . . . at least not that they confided in me.

I have a few theories on why I wanted chemotherapy. The first is most likely . . . that I want to do anything possible to aid my survival. As awful as it is, chemotherapies, especially for some breast cancers, have proven amazingly effective over the years and I want in on that success. My 79 year-old neighbor had breast cancer, mastectomy, chemotherapy and radiation 25 years ago. Although she is failing in memory, she still recounts with revulsion her chemotherapy sessions – and how her son had to talk her into the last two rounds when she wanted to give up. And she's still HERE to remember it . . . wanting new boobs, because the ones reconstructed 25 years ago are not as perky. I want that (not the boob part – the survival part). If Dr. Lifeline wants me to do chemotherapy every year to stay here on this Earth, with my husband and helping David reach his full potential, I will.

Part of me was fearful that I wouldn't get chemotherapy and was trying arguments in my mind as to why I should get it. What if the nodes sampled were not engaged, *but*, there were nodes not taken that were. Even before I was told that I needed therapy, I wanted it to catch any "floating" cancer cells that may not be apparent. If I needed to swallow a flame-thrower to do that, I swear I'd try.

I think the dark part of me sees chemotherapy as a fitting punishment for not catching the lump sooner. Despite the yearly mammograms, I should have found it sooner. Going through "CHEMO" would teach me to be more vigilant, to be more careful, to . . . punish myself for getting cancer.

And it would be punishing. Among the best advice I received from Karen Angel were two instructions, one which helped me physically and the other mentally. The first was to drink water like crazy to minimize the effects of chemotherapy. For the day before each round, the day of and two days after, Karen said to drink the equivalent of two 2-liter bottles of water a day. The chemotherapy would do its thing, but to minimize damage to the good tissues and minimize side effects, washing the excess out of my body would help.

The second was to set up a monthly calendar, documenting how I felt and any side effects. Round __, Day 1 through Day 21 on a calendar large enough to write on. By mapping the side effects and recognizing the worst days, Karen said that, after the first Round, I could truly lay those 21 days over the 21 days for following Rounds, plan for the worst days and the best days and could live my life with a game plan. I planned to work from home when I was immuno-suppressed and from work when I rebounded, school functions on good days, days Thanksgiving and Halloween on rebound days, etc.. Plan A, Plan B, Plan C to Plan D . . . Chemothera-py.

September 5, 2012

"I can't believe I'm going to have chemotherapy today," I thought. I ran my hand along my left collarbone, feeling the alien port just under the skin. It itched and pulled and, even five days later, I slept worse with the port than I had even since the mastectomies. It ached and felt foreign – like I was a real-life "Manchurian Candidate".

Yesterday, I had broken down and truly sobbed. In front of my sweet husband and in front of Karen Angel, before whom I tried to be so strong. She had taken Bill and me on a tour through the Infusion Therapy center, across the Cancer Center waiting room from oncology, so we would prepare as well as we could for today and know what to expect. Walking through the infusion clinic was heart-rending . . . horrifying that I would be treated there tomorrow, inspiring in the quiet strength of those receiving treatment, overwhelming that there were so many (so, so many). Every chair was full. I walked out and into the hall. Karen asked if we had questions or needed any information and I had lost it and couldn't articulate why. Karen hugged me as Bill stood by, both worried and confused, and I choked out "there are so many" and couldn't say more.

The tour did prepare me somewhat for today, at least in mind-set. I packed a little bag with water, chapstick, lotion, a magazine, my phones (planning to work on my Blackberry as long as I could), snacks. Bill packed a BIG bag for himself, more water, books (still working on his Doctorate in Executive Leadership), many more snacks . . . it's like we were going on a world trek instead of spending the next five hours in Infusion Therapy. How to prepare.

Bill pulled up out front and left the car running, while he came to the door to pick me up. He had dropped the Buddy off at school this morning and my therapy started at 9:00. If everything went as planned, we would be home in time to pick him up from school. I had been warned that the first round of chemotherapy took longer than the others as they ran each medicine slowly, watching for adverse effects and allergic reactions. If I wasn't finished in time, Bill would pick up the Buddy and they would both come and pick me up with David being told I just had an appointment.

Bill gently loaded me into the care with our collective luggage and drove the short distance to the Cancer Center. We parked and walked in, holding hands silently, facing this new hurdle together. I had worn stretchy pants due both to my need to pee frequently (drinking 4 liters of water daily) and lack of strength and mobility in pulling my pants up. I also wore a loose-fitting tank and unbuttoned blouse over top, not knowing how warm or cold I'd be. I wanted to be comfortable, to give easy access to my port, but hide it at the same time.

I signed into the Infusion Therapy window at the opposite side from Oncology and sat down, not knowing where to look or what to think. The television hanging from the wall was on a morning show from some nation station, but the talking-heads could have been talking Greek for all I could comprehend. I was seriously sinking into a funk while Bill thumbed his Blackberry – oblivious to my growing panic. Suddenly, I heard the rumble of light laughter around the room at something said on the television. I looked for the source and found both patients (some without hair) and supporters, chuckling and watching television like in any waiting room. It was one of the most beautiful sounds I have ever heard . . . laughter in an oncology waiting room. The reaffirmation that life will go on and can be enjoyed and you can laugh, even in the face of Chemotherapy. The stone rolled off of my shoulders enough that I sat a little higher and breathed a little lighter. I found myself looking around the room in a way I hadn't before.

The nurse called us into Infusion and led Bill and me down the corridor to my spot. Karen Angel was there waiting. There was an armchair and guest chair in a small, curtained bay with a little cabinet on one side and IV stand on the other. The nurse goes through her questions pre-procedure and really listens to my responses. She examines my bruised collarbone where the port is and asks when I had it installed. "Friday", I said. Her wince was barely perceptible as she asked if I put the numbing cream on it this morning to lessen the discomfort of accessing the port. I hadn't – deliberately. Karen Angel and I discussed how precious the port is and to minimize contaminations or access to it for other than chemotherapy. I have decide to not use the crème and to only use it for therapy, not to draw blood from to minimize the risk of infection. As Karen holds one hand, Bill holds the other, as the nurse accesses my port for the first time, saying "one, two and three" to let me know when I can expect. It hurt a bit, but nothing like I'd already experiences. The nurse sees a good return of blood back into the tube, so we know it's functioning.

I had feared the moment when these cancer-killing, life-giving, toxic chemicals entered my body. I was apprehensive that I'd feel a burn or something to let me know. It was nothing like that. It was better and worse. It wasn't painful for me and didn't immediately make me sick. What it did, though, was slowly erase my mind as *the medicine entered my body. Little by little, the edges around my world got fuzzier and I felt like I was thinking through mud.*

Karen Angel had prepared me for that and that I'd get myself back by the next time, but that each round I may get less back and more slowly. The analogy she used was that of me in a boat on a lake. As the chemicals enter my body, they push me across the lake into the fog to the other shore. As the days pass, I drink a lot of water to rid me of excess and I rest, she and Dr. Lifeline and his team slowly pull me back through the fog to the near shore. With each round, they push me out again and there is more fog to come back through. I hate losing my mind each time, but I'm not afraid. Karen Angel assures me that, even when I'm too tired to help row and keep the boat steady, she, Dr. Lifeline and his team – my team – all have their hands under my boat, keeping me afloat until my last journey when I safely reach the near shore for good.

September 26, 2012
October 17, 2012
November 7, 2012
November 28, 2012
December 19, 2012

Friends – Earthbound Angels

It's an interesting observation to see how people act around someone who has a cancer diagnosis. Some treat you with kid gloves, as if you are disabled (no "handicapped sticker" needed or wanted here), some ask personal questions that they would never otherwise ask (did you get really constipated post-surgery) and still others run from the sight of you. The latter group is slightly disappointing for the few whom I've known for years. Believe me, the last thing I want to talk about is cancer, so I'm not going to be the downer going into excruciating detail. A normal conversation about sports, the weather, the school, the kids, work, food, etc. is just fine. I do cut them some slack, though. Although I've not been at a loss for words when others have gone through illnesses, I know that some folks are uncomfortable with illness and don't know what to say. I, for one, will know that I am again "well" and normal when folks stop asking how I'm doing and how I'm feeling. It's well meaning, but a constant reminder of the battle that I feel I have won. Lord willing.

I've never been one to have a large gaggle of girlfriends. I'm not good at keeping up with friends who don't live near (other than with one or two) and don't even have a Facebook account. I'm one of *those*. If I want to know something about someone, I'll ask. If I want them to know something, I'll pick up the phone, send an e-mail or, most often, text them. I watch in awe of those who have different clutches of friends . . . a high school group to have drinks with or a former co-workers group to meet for drinks or a "our kids were in daycare together" group for Sunday potluck. I don't have that knack.

What I have been blessed with is a small group of really trusted friends, neighbors and friends of my husband, who have made a world of difference in this scorched-Earth world of Cancer. My friends at work sent so much food post-mastectomy that Bill and I didn't need to worry about cooking for weeks (not that I had much appetite). They facilitated my working from home on the days that I was at my nadir in immune-suppression (the low point, when I'm most vulnerable to germs), and acted as gate-keepers to the consumption that can be my job.

Bill's best friends were also champions . . . hugs from Eva, motivation from Tom and Brenda (who herself is a 15+ year Survivor), and companionship from Bruce, who would get Bill out of the house from time to time. Then there are the McGees . . . their two sons are around David's age (and who led by example in Orthodontics). Brad sat with Bill during my marathon surgery, came to the hospital to visit me and would occasionally call just to "check in." Jennifer (who also created the beautiful cover art for this book) brought over pre-made dinners to put in the freezer and a great breakfast casserole. Never prying, never pitying, just . . . there.

During the lowest of lows, when I barely had the energy to get off of the couch and my thoughts were foggier than San Francisco, invariably, Melissa would show up at our door with a full dinner . . . salad, bread, entrée and dessert . . . all homemade and beautifully made with little post-prep needed. Rachel would likewise, lamenting the fact that she (like I) generally order and pick-up and "I bet that Melissa homemade hers. Well, it's the thought that counts." I love Rachel – she says what she thinks and she loves Melissa, too, so she was bitching the way good friends do who know their strengths and admire strengths in others. For the record, Rachel owns the absolute best bakery with gourmet cupcakes and pies. Baking *is* her thing, even if cooking is not.

Another friend, Katy, my longest in Charleston and the editor of this tome', would send frequent e-mails of support, normal Mother frustrations, worries and school laments, and would leave flowers or goodies on the doorstep. Katy insisted upon our adding her to the school permitted "pick ups" for David. Her beautiful girls go to the same elementary and she wanted to make sure we had back ups in case Bill and I couldn't get to David for some reason. Great girl.

Then there is Deanna. She is as blunt as they come, but there is no one with a bigger heart. She "mothers" full-out and has the uncanny ability to read my mind. On a Monday, five days after my first round of chemotherapy, Bill was scheduled to attend a business golf outing out of town. It was early September, the weather was perfect and he hadn't left my side for an hour in the past two months. He had awoken the Saturday morning, before, tearful and fretful . . . "I'm not going," he said. "I'll just call and tell them that I can't make it." I protested and stuck to my guns, insisting that I was and would be fine. Inside, I was terrified.

Bill called "Helga" and told her that he was going to be out of town. True to fashion, Deanna said "I'm not doing anything. I'll pick up some pizza and come over Monday after work." Also, not-surprisingly, she showed up that Saturday afternoon to take my emotional temperature. Bill was outside with David and she looked at me and said, "you know, David is not going to find you dead on Monday with Bill out of town. You're going to be fine." I hadn't said a word . . . not a word! Her sister had found her father when she was eigth years old, and maybe that enhanced her perception. Maybe just that she knows me so well . . . my only true fears in battling this illness are all wrapped up in David. She knew that my fear on Monday was that I would have an adverse reaction to the chemical cocktail and my son would find me. Tears running down my face, my throat too tight to speak, I simply nodded. And her giving voice to my fears somehow lessened them.

Not only did Deanna come over for dinner on Monday, but she ran over during lunch to check on me. Since picking the Buddy up from school that afternoon was my first time driving in two months, she suggested that I put a pillow between my stomach and the seatbelt to keep it off of both the port and the dratted expanders. She offered to pick him up, but I knew that I couldn't let myself feel disabled – or let David see me as such.

Deanna called me as she was leaving work and asked about the pizza. "No need," I told her, "my neighbor, Melissa, dropped off some chicken and wild rice, salad and cobbler with ice cream." When Deanna got to our house, she popped the chicken into the oven for the specified time and set the table. As we sat down to eat she asked, "how good a cook is Melissa?" I said, "you be the judge." We tucked into an awesome meal, agreeing on how fabulous it was. "What does Melissa look like?" she asked. "Beautiful," I responded, "thin and she is smart and so nice that you can't hate her for being pretty"." She looked at me and said, "what a bitch." I laughed and told her that that's what Rachel says.

Hair, Hair, Hair – Here There and Everywhere

Interestingly, despite the ravages that chemotherapy can and does wage on your body while it's doing its thing, the one people focus on the most is the hair loss. Maybe because that is the most visible manifestation of the war being raged for survival. Maybe because it's such a stark contrast to the average person seen while walking down the street . . . especially for women. Most women have hair. I'm not sure why that is the focus because that's the least of your worries.

As I've written, I've never been a hair person. That doesn't mean it made losing it any easier. For me, it wasn't about the vanity or loss, but about logistics. Ever the Type A, I wanted to make sure I was prepared and had a game plan . . . mostly for the Buddy's sake. Even though the belief is that children with Asperger's (or on the Autism Spectrum in general) aren't as empathetic, loving or compassionate as "normal" children. I can't speak for all families as no two Aspies are any more alike than anyone else. I can attest that David is incredibly loving and gets so worried when he sees anyone in distress. He didn't (and doesn't) know what cancer is or that his Momma had it. He did know "surgery" and played, worried, on my bed for weeks after. I knew that, if he saw me bald, he'd never get over it. He'd question and worry, and worry. I've had loving, well-learned friends advise that he'd be fine seeing me without hair if we explained that it was part of my medicine and would get used to it. That wasn't going to happen.

The day before I got the port installed, Deanna drove me down to a place nearby called "Resolutions 2" a store for folks with many issues that need the pick-me-up and focus on the aesthetics that can restore a sense of peace and normalcy in shattered lives. We went down primarily to find a bra with some breast inserts so I could wear something as my expanders were filled. The secondary goal was to look at wigs and head coverings for the certain hair loss coming my way. Deanna had heard about Resolutions 2 from another girlfriend of hers (now a girlfriend of mine, Donna) so she made an appointment and off we went.

Pulling into the parking lot, you know it is someplace special. The curb in front of the store is pink and the parking spaces adorned with painted pink ribbons like you would see for a handicapped-parking space. Walking in, it looks, feels and smells like a spa or salon with the bonus of a wall of wigs in styles much more trendy and fashionable than I've been able to muster with my own real hair.

After the bra and boob fitting and purchase (man, I had forgotten how heavy boobs were), Deanna and I browsed the wall of wigs. Instead of looking for hairstyles that matched what I had, I looked for a short style for which I could get my own hair cut to match before it started falling out. My theory was that It would be easier to hide hair loss of shorter hair than long. The owner, who founded her store as a hair loss client herself, frustrated that the only selections in the valley were hairpieces made for me, was so knowledgeable about wig materials, hair composition, fit, etc.. She advised not to try on or buy right then as the hair fits differently on a bald head than it does one with hair. I was impressed that she wasn't so anxious to make an additional few hundred dollars on by selling a wig to me on the spot, but she and everyone at Resolutions 2 truly take the clients into account.

With the hair style in mind of the wig I intended to purchase, I went to our family salon. I got a short pixie cut the day before my first round of chemotherapy. Sitting in the chair, I explained to our stylist, who hadn't seen me since before diagnosis and surgery, what I wanted and why. To his credit, for such a young man, he didn't give me the "pity look", but carefully guided me over to the sinks, and gently laid my back, mindful of my achy, newly-installed port, and gave me the best cut I've ever had.

After my first round of chemotherapy, my hair didn't start falling out until almost the end of the third week, right before the second round. It started as a few more hairs in the brush, then a few more in the drain. Then, during that third week, I could run my hand through my hair and come away with a handful. More and more and more. I knew it was time to take matters into my own hands. Three weeks after I'd visited Resolutions 2 with Deanna, my sweet husband and I dropped the Buddy off for school and headed back to the shop.

We had made an appointment with the stylist on staff at Resolutions 2. Although a lot of her job entails freshening up styles on the wigs purchased and restoring some of the hair pieces to their original luster, Donna had had the stylist buzz her hair off when she was losing it during her chemotherapy the year before. Walking in, I felt no nerves, but was really ready to take control of this side-effect. I showed Bill a couple of the styles that Deanna and I had looked at during our visit, and he liked both, especially the one that was identical to my new haircut. We brought that wig from the wall of wigs into the salon.

Back in the salon area of Resolutions 2, I sat in the chair while Bill sat in the "guest chair" at the other end. The stylist, a mid-thirties, pretty woman, closed the salon door for some privacy, laid her hands on my shoulders and asked to make sure I was ready for her to shave my head. Bill and I assured her that I was ready and I said that I preferred to take charge of losing my hair rather than to wait for it to come out naturally, which would take weeks. My establishing the timing also somehow let me feel that I was in control over my treatment and my prognosis – that I was doing something rather than being a victim and having it "done" to me. The stylist nodded in understanding. She was a cancer survivor herself (gynecological, not breast) so really understood.

She asked if I wanted to watch or wait until the end and I told her to spin me around from the mirror. She nodded again and quickly got to work. Bill chatted with her while she buzzed, I stayed largely silent, anticipating my bald head . . . my "chemotherapy patient" head. When she finished and dusted me off, she said "you have a nice head. Are you ready?" Although I don't know if "ready" was the right word, I said that I was. Spinning me toward the mirror, I looked up . . . and really didn't look that different. I looked like me without hair. Bill laughed gently, "G.I. Jane" he said, smiling at my reflection. He got up and gave me a kiss in his special way . . . making me feel like I'm the most beautiful woman on the planet.

The stylist rubbed some lotion on my scalp and put a nylon cap on my head to try on the wig "for sanitary reasons". No one tries on wigs without the head condom. The hair piece had a flesh-colored, latex crown that the hair was sewn into, so putting it on, it looked like my scalp, not a weave of hair. Amazingly, the style matched my new haircut, now on-the-floor-haircut, perfectly. Bill and I took before and after pictures and it really was uncanny. The Buddy would never know. The stylist brought an asymmetrical style in for me to try on, too. She said it was her favorite and popular, and recounted how one of the clients referred to it as "ass-symetrical" and laughed. I tried that on and loved it, too. At Bill's urging, I bought both, totaling about $500 – cringe-worthy, but that way I'd have a spare while one was drying from being washed or if one was damaged. After buying the care shampoos and pick, I left wearing one and carrying the other and two wig-forms out. I also picked up a hat and two nighttime head covers. The stylist said that, despite how hot it was this first week in September, my head would get cold at night without hair. Love Resolutions 2.

Throughout my hairless months, I fell into a routine. While it was still hot outside, other than when I was with David, I generally just had a cap on my head or scarf at work or going to appointments . . . or nothing if it was one of the days I was working from home. Even though modern wigs are really comfortable mesh scalp pieces into which the hair is sewn, making it lighter and cooler, wearing hair is still hotter than having hair. I'd put my hair on right before school ended, so the Buddy didn't know a thing. In the mornings, when I'd get up to make his lunch or snack, or on the weekends, I'd keep a towel on my head as if I'd just gotten out of the shower, or I'd put on hair before he got up. At night, after David was in bed, I'd either wrap a towel around my head or one of the nightcaps.

As the weather grew cooler, then cold, I'd wear one of the wigs all the time. They were just warmer than going without. I'd wash the one I was wearing every three or four days, soaking it in the wig shampoo in cool water in the sink, patting it dry and resetting it on the wig form to dry until its turn again, and would rotate the wigs that way. Even though the pixie and "ass-symmetrical" styles are different, the Buddy didn't appear to notice. Both styles are short and, well, he is male after all. The most challenging weeks were during Thanksgiving and Christmas breaks where he was home all the time. I was extra careful to wear hair all the time.

Aside from the head hair loss was another concept that I didn't think about beforehand. Head hair isn't the only hair that falls out. For the first time in three decades, I didn't need to shave my legs. The very few hairs that stayed in my legs were fine and light and not noticeable. The hair on my arms fell out, my eyebrows got really thin (thank God Resolutions 2 had eyebrow makeup) as did hair "down there". Crazy. Hadn't even considered it. Bill called me the "Mexican hairless" for the breed of cat that has no coat.

I did manage to keep my eyelashes throughout the entire six rounds of chemotherapy and for a month after. Then, just as my hair was starting to really come in and I felt that I had turned the "hair corner", my eyelashes all fell out. Added insult to injury. For a few weeks, I tried to wear false eyelashes, trying the different styles available on the makeup shelves. Really, who knows that there are many styles of eyelash other than one of the Real Housewives of . . . ? David quickly put the cabbosh on the false eyelashes, though. He kept staring at them and finally said, "Mom, your eyelashes are too shiny. I don't like them." I told him that I had cut mine to try false ones like the ladies on TV and he said, "grow yours back and don't do that again." Lord willing, Buddy, Momma won't need to.

Interestingly, every few months my eyelashes fall out again. Not all, but most. I read somewhere where you constantly shed eyelashes, but just a few every once in a while, and they grow back until ready to fall out again. Since they are on a different cycle, most of the time, people aren't wholly lash-less. I guess since mine all fell out at the same time, they are now on the same cycle. Not sure if that is the reason, but it does make sense.

For anyone who wonders about hair regrowth, average rate is about one-half an inch per month. Mine is a little faster. It started growing back in a month after my last cycle and I had my pixie back four months later. My hair is almost entirely gray and likely had been for years. My Dad had gone gray in his early 30s, so I took after him for that. Mother is 70 and still has very few grays. For some reason, the gray bothered me when the hairless part did not. I had it colored immediately when I had enough hair to make it worthwhile. For a hair color role-model, I looked to Charlize Theron, who had buzzed her hair for a movie and who was a little more than a month ahead of me for regrowth. Although I don't resemble her, I admire the gracious way she handled regrowth . . . light-brown stubble, darker inch-or-so, dark blonde as it grew, then back to her blonde. It was flattering on her and gave me a pattern to follow which, I believe, worked for me, too.

And if anyone is wondering about regrowth of hair elsewhere, I can report on that. Leg hair grows five times as fast as head hair – at least for me. I had been shaving for a month before I had discernable head hair to speak of. One of my nurses in Radiation Therapy (herself a 9 year Survivor post-chemotherapy) said that she only had one hair grow back on her legs in all the years since. Showing it to me, she said she kept it as a reminder of what she went through. Arm hair was about the same rate as head hair. Pubic hair, for me, grew three times as fast. I didn't have the mobility to wax or shave closely in the early months, so I definitely was a little more "Welcome Back Kotter" than I had ever been for a while. In case anyone was wondering.

The Commodification of Cancer

Like many who have had cancer, I avoid any reminders of the illness. In the last year since my diagnosis, I'm only now starting to be able to read the obituaries again. Even so, I only read the name and scan the list of family so I can send a card or flowers. I don't want to know how old they were or see the words "after a courageous battle with cancer." I just can't. I flip the channel for an episode of any show on rerun where I know it's a death episode or cancer. And children's movies, particularly the animated ones, typically have the hero or heroine losing their mother, father or both. You'd think these writers would be more creative.

I don't know if it's my newly acquired sensitivity to cancer or if my perception is reality, but there seem to be many commercials about cancer treatment centers on now. Instead of a referral from a trusted doctor or knowing that a particular hospital or center provides excellent care, marketers have packaged cancer treatment like car commercials, showing the shiny, latest model. It bugs me. If there is anything that shouldn't be commercialized it is cancer treatment.

Faith, Angels and Hearing God

In the earliest days post-diagnosis, post-surgery and during chemotherapy, I was desolate. I'd wait for Bill to take David to school some mornings, barely able to contain myself, and scream and sob during the time that he was gone. Not every day, but a few times a week most definitely. Not asking "why me", as to do so questions God's will, but in fear and sadness of the new reality I was stuck in.

I have always talked to God throughout the day even just a "thank you, God" when the traffic lights roll my way when I'm late for a meeting. Definitely a "please, Lord, let the Buddy be his best self today" in the mornings before school. And, invariably, when I read about someone who has been hurt, I immediately pray for healing and comfort, as well as for families who have lost loved ones. I realized that I also need to thank God for each day that I've not been promised. None of us are promised another day, but going through cancer has reinforced that for me. I'm thankful for every day.

Invariably, when I'd bottom out, I would be given Godly comfort. I know that God *does* answer every prayer, but sometimes the answer is "no." There is one prayer that God always grants and that is for peace and comfort. Even in my agony and fear, when I've prayed for peace in my heart, I have felt the grace of peace given. Every time. And there has been more.

Bill said that when his brother, Dave, was battling cancer, he'd sit under the trees and just stare at them. When asked what he was looking at, Dave had responded "angels." I, too, have seen during the worst of times. Maybe it's like thestrals in Potter stories where only those who have seen death those magical creatures. Only way better – only those who are in true need and ask for comfort can see angels. I know most aren't going to believe this, and others may chalk it up to wishful thinking on my part, but I know in my heart that they were there. Like Dave, I would see them shimmering on the tops of the trees, winking and glowing, keeping sentry over my heart and others. They didn't have wings, but appeared as slivers of light in the trees across the street . . . on the opposite side of the leave to where the sun would shine. Although I no longer see them, I know they are there.

There are other reassurances as well. When we pulled into the beach house at Kure Beach this year, I was momentarily overcome with emotion. Happiness to be there with my family, anguish over all that we'd gone through since the last trip, fear of whether this would be my last trip to our family sanctuary . . . I was frozen in the front seat, afraid to get out. As Bill opened his door to start unloading, music from a radio across the street was blaring "Stronger" by Kelly Clarkson . . . my chemotherapy anthem. Hearing it gave me the courage to get out of the car and start carrying.

As we brought the first load up, we walked out onto the deck to look at the ocean. Out on the water I saw the last of a rainbow, from a dissipating storm out at sea. Rainbows have always been one of my favorite images from the Bible – God's promise. Seeing the rainbow and hearing my chemo anthem immediately gave me peace

Even random signs I believe are God sent. I bottomed out emotionally in November of this year, 2013. I just felt tired and lousy and sad. I woke up with that ever present tug of survival in my head – the "how long would it be before cancer returns and I sip on the chemo cocktail again" even though I shouldn't need to do it again. Don't get me wrong – I'll do it yearly if it means I get to watch my son grow up, I'd like to watch him grow up without chemotherapy assistance, thank you very much. This particular morning, I was really low. I heard the "do-da-do" from my phone, indicating that I'd received a text. It was from the Twitterverse. One of the random searcher ran across my Twitter bio, that I had changed to say "Breast Cancer Survivor (love saying that)" and the tweet had copied it from my bio and simply said "right on." I smiled, the weight of the world rolled off of my shoulders and I thanked God for this day that I've not been promise and thanked Him for needing reinforcement. I'm grateful that He understands when I'm weak. Although trusting His will, I sometimes need reassurance – I think we all do. These little nuggets out of nowhere are God speaking to me. I know they are.

I believe I will survive cancer. Even if I don't, God has me and is in control. He will take care of David and give Bill the comfort and strength that he will need. I just hope it never comes to that.

December 19, 2012

Tired, battle-weary, but ready. Today is my sixth and final round of chemotherapy. Lord willing. My numbers remain good from bloodwork throughout, so I haven't needed to postpone any therapy session to wait for my numbers to rebound. Karen Angel had told me that, even though the fatigue would be overwhelming at this point, as it compounds from round to round, I'd be so elated with reaching the end that I wouldn't notice it as much.

"Is it the end?", I wondered, the same question that I'd be asking myself throughout. "Will I ever be rid of this nightmare? Will I ever return to "normal" again?" Not the relatively care-free, unburdened normal that I was before – I appreciated the new level of empathy that my journey had given me. I thought more, felt more, reached out more. No longer would I think, "I need to send ___ a note" and then not follow through . . . I followed through, realizing how much the small gestures meant to me over these past 6 months. Six months – a lifetime ago. A "different Beth" ago. An "I can't believe this is my reality" ago.

I hadn't slept much last night. I rarely sleep at all anymore, actually. Although never a Kelsey Grammer fan, I've relied on repeats of "Frazier" during those endless, insomniac nights. It was only when I was beyond exhaustion that I could fall asleep. I had stayed up even longer than usual last night, crying and planning. I'm both overjoyed that this is my last chemotherapy and frightened that it won't be my last . . . that I'll need to revisit again in the future for more clean-up . . . or to extend my life. Karen Angel had said that she has patients dance out of therapy and through the waiting room in celebration and motivation for all. I listened to my "anthem" over and over last night, sobbing with fear, relief and hope. "Stronger" by Kelly Clarkson, is mine. Someone had sent to me a link to a YouTube posted by the Hemoncology Floor of Seattle Children's Hospital, of their young patient warriors, caregivers and medical staff signing "Stronger" in definance of their illnesses. The blessing that it was me and not my Buddy going through this was not lost on me. The song also resonated with me that I AM a stronger Beth than before cancer and December 20, 2012 is "just my beginning."

I had sent an e-mail to family on both sides the night before, sharing my Anthem and my joy . . .

"Last round today ... last bag hung in last round. They truly don't expect me to be back - as my Advocate says, you are going to survive this and more on with your life. Please God ...

The tradition for those of us fortunate to get into a Therapy Trials and have my Advocate is that we get to dance out of our last therapy. Sharing my Anthem with you in the YouTube below - please know you're with me while I dance. I love you all - and "thank you"."

Late night sobbing notwithstanding, I bolted out of bed, singing "Stronger" in my head. Bill has had a bad chest cold (more than the "Man-cold") for the past couple of days, so we'd decided that he wouldn't accompany me to this last round. We couldn't risk exposing the other immuno-suppressed warriors in the waiting room and therapy to whatever ick he had. The only one he's missed is this last one and I know it's weighing on him.

Bill was up having hot coffee, trying to loosen his chest congestion. I got the Buddy into and out of his bath, me with a towel on my own head, hiding the baldness. He remained oblivious and I determined to keep him that way. I shoed David downstairs where he made his nest in front of the TV, watching his morning show while eating cereal. Bill set out his clothes while I went back upstairs, and, in between sips of water, put on hair, layer clothes over my scarred and expander-stretched body and draw on eyebrows and put on make-up.

Still sipping as I was coming downstairs, I said, "Miss Deanna is going to pick up Mom for a work meeting in a few minutes, Buddy", so he wouldn't think it strange that Mom is leaving before he is. Deanna was picking me up and would drop me off for therapy, to collect me again when I called her. "Ok Mom," he replied, bounding up to keep watch at the door (in his underwear) for Miss Deanna, one of his favorite people, never mind that she wouldn't be there for another 20 minutes.

I went into the kitchen to pack his lunch and snack, checked off his homework and signed the planner and packed it off into his commando backpack. Bill was helping the Buddy get dressed, taking his allergy medicine and brushing his teeth. As usual, Deanna pulled into the driveway early. My son threw the front door open and yelled "Hello, Miss Deanna!!!" and bounced back into the house. I grabbed my purse, my bag of rations and work and turned to Bill. With tears in his eyes, he pulled me into a gentle, but firm hug, holding me, holding us together for a moment longer before my last descent. "I've got the Buddy," he said, "thank Deanna for me" as he waved to her.

In the car and on our way, there was no need for small talk. Other than her words of encouragement (gasp) and logistical planning, we didn't talk much at all. Getting signed in at the Infusion Therapy window, I handed over some fresh baked goods, expressing thanks for their loving, excellent care along with my best wishes for them. I can't imagine what they see . . . how they survive it emotionally.

I was taken back to therapy timely, as they have the routine down to an art, and directed into my recliner in cubby I hadn't been in previously. While they were getting my meds sorted, I took a quick trip to the bathroom, hoping to cut down on one tethered trip during my 4 or so hours here. Drinking four liters of water a day is work. Settling back in, my Infusion Nurse for this last round greated me with the standard questions. Meds, trips to the ER, any unexpected health issues to report, feel like hurting myself, exposure to violence, etc.. Satisfied with my responses, she readied the needle connector to my port. Karen Angel popped around the corner at that moment to check on my. As she did for the first round in accessing my port, she held my hand for this final round until I was hooked up and taped down.

"Where's Bill," she asked, sitting down in the "guest chair" after the nurse had left to attend her next in a day's line of patients. "Chest crud," I said, "we didn't want to expose anyone." She nodded. "That's wise. I know today means a lot to him, but he's being considerate to other patients and their families. And you. Are you staying away from him?" I told her that I was as David had been sleeping with Daddy for a couple of months instead of me, both so I didn't need to worry about getting kicked or elbowed in the expanders at night, but to minimize my proximity contact with anyone who may be harboring a bug.

We talked a bit about our families, my journey, getting on with life and affirmed that God is in control. Having an Advocate who shares the same spiritual beliefs has been such a blessing. Never waivering in faith and perspective, she shores me up when the water is lashing my shores. "I still can't believe your numbers," she said, referring to my bloodwork results two days prior. Throughout the onslaught, while my red bloodcell count, white bloodcell count, etc., dipped dramatically, I still didn't bottom out or even need the Neulasta white blood cell booster shot throughout. It's a good thing, since my insurance carrier was draconian over not letting me have it, even with Dr. Lifeline. calling personally and insisting it was protocol.

During my fourth round bloodwork, when Karen Angel and I had looked at it while waiting for my Dr. Lifeline. exam, I had expressed my concerns about my counts being so low. "What happens if it's not working for me?" I worried. "Maybe I'm not bottoming out because it's not strong enough." She looked at me, held my hand up to me, showing me the Muehrcke's on my nails extending the entire breadth of the nails. These stripes, like rings on a tree trunk, mark the assault to my body. The acid reflux, kidney aches, night sweats, hair loss, "chemo brain" . . . all of it assures us that it is strong enough. "God is carrying me through then," I said, knowing that it is the explanation. "I've never seen anything like it," she had said, nodding.

Now for this final round, she reminded me that I needed to say "good-bye" to my medical staff in Infusion Therapy when I leave and before we dance out. "You should not ever see them in here again," she assured me. I knew, "for this kind of cancer" and "Lord willing" were not spoken. It still helped. "My prognosis is excellent", I remind myself often and did so as she stood up to go to check on her other charges, promising to stop in before I finished. Today, as my mind slowly was turning to mush, as the boggy layers of muck rolled through and I started going down the rabbit hole, I put the fears aside and imagined the chemical army taking aim at whatever alien invaders may still be in my body. I prayed for peace and strength and then let it go.

In no time, it seemed, I was ready to be unhooked for the last time. The bag changes had gone smoothly, I only needed two tethered trips to the bathroom, pushing my IV bag as I went, and had gotten the majority of thank you cards finished, from the literally hundreds of cards, noted, gifts and contacts I had received. No matter how lousy I had felt, I tried to do a few every day so as to not get overwhelmed. Like clockwork (the nurse must have called her) Karen Angel popped down to watch the final unloading. I texted Deanna that I would be discharged shortly so she could start her trek as well.

"Are you ready to dance, Sweet Friend?" Karen Angel said, smiling her magnificent smile. I had sent the link to "Stronger" to her so she knew my Anthem. "Say 'good-bye' to everyone, because they won't be seeing you in here again." I did as she instructed, as tears started to flow. The nurses, familiar with this routine and with Karen, smiled, waved and wished me well and hoped to see me "outside" sometime. I scooped up my bags, Karen Angel grabbed my hand and raised it in triumph as I started singing to the tune in my head "Stronger". Karen hummed along as we wound our way out of Infusion Therapy, with "thumbs up" from my fellow warriors, out through the waiting room of both therapy and oncology and through to the oncology side for my final release to the rest of my life. I hope others found

strength in my awful singing and tear-streaked dance. I hope we gave them a laugh at these two middle-aged women, crying and boogying through the Cancer Center, oblivious to everything but the moment . . . the celebration. I hope.

When we finished, Karen Angel walked me out to the front curb in front of the building. Predictably, Deanna was there, front row, standing beside the car with her beatific smile shining. Neither woman had met the other, but knew the other through me and stepped into a full, kindred hug of friendship and mutual respect. "You e-mail me every day. Every Day," Karen said as she always did, while Deanna helped me into the car. As we drove away, Deanna asked, "so did you dance?"

"Oh yeah," I responded and recounted the last journey to her while she drove me home.

I had texted Bill that we were on our way, so he was standing on the front step, looking awful, when we pulled up. As Deanna helped me out of her car, he burst into tears and hugged me, crying in relief and sorrow that he hadn't been able to come with me. He hugged Helga, too, and thanked her again for her friendship and support. Ever modest and impatient over accolades she waved us off, jumped back into her car and rode off.

My boys and I settled into the last trip to the opposite shore, with Christmas around the corner and gifts bought pre-chemo. Having the last round of therapy behind us was the greatest gift. That portion of my journey is over, Lord willing, with radiation and years of drug therapy to follow.

Despair and Desperation

When checking into my oncology check-ups, I fill out the "stress scale" setting forth my level of distress and ticking off some of the areas that may be a concern. A lot of the issues I worry about aren't on the checklist, but I can't put into words my exact area of distress. When I look at the scale, I usually find my stress level relatively low. Breast cancer, notwithstanding, I <u>know</u> I am blessed and remain relatively peaceful. Not that I don't understand despair.

One question the Infusion Therapy professionals ask before they hook you up to chemotherapy is "have you thought about hurting yourself?" The first time I heard the question, I looked at Karen Angel and said, "really? I'm here to save my life, why would I do anything to shorten it?" She just nodded without saying anything.

As the months have gone by, with every setback and every health concern and every false alarm, I start to understand more why that question is asked. I doubt that the interviewee would give an honest answer to that question, but I'm glad it's asked. I marvel at those patients who are deemed "terminal" and how some of them just get on with their lives, for however long they have. We're all, "terminal" though, aren't we . . . God doesn't promise us another day and death is certain, no matter the cause. I hope if I am not the ultimate victor in this battle, I can exemplify courage for other as others, like Mary Sue, did for me. I would want my family to be proud of me and for the Buddy to know that I didn't leave this Earth or him one minute before I had to.

I would be lying, though if I didn't admit to understanding and empathizing with those who I know choose to hasten their journey. Illness is torture without true end, at least psychologically. Treatment is painful, mind-losing, undignified without guarantee of success. I read the stories about sufferers committing suicide when receiving news about diagnosis or relapse. I cry with relief and agony, empathetic as to both, when I hear about a decades' devoted spouse ending the other spouse's life who was suffering with a disease with no hope of ever ending. They love their spouse and want to end suffering more than they love themselves and wanting to keep that love close forever.

The one story that really struck me was the woman somewhere in the Midwest who had received a Breast Cancer diagnosis. She killed her teen-aged children, her husband and herself. I didn't dive into the story, wanting to protect her, somehow, from curiosity-seeking into a desperation so profound – wanting to protect myself from seeing if her diagnosis was similar to mine. In my horror and sorrow, though, was an understanding of the hope-crushing word "cancer" that, for some, there is nothing else needed to push them over the cliff. While I wouldn't dream of depriving the world of my David and what amazing things he will accomplish (I'm hopeful cancer will be only discussed in textbooks by then), I do understand a Mother's despair of imagining her children's agony at her loss. I get that – for any of us, particularly Mothers, to say that we *don't* get that would be an untruth. Or they are unwilling to vocalize that deep, dark fear of leaving our children before we know they are set, on the right path and largely self-sufficient.

If any of you are reading this and feel that despair, that desperation so vividly that you can't see out of the darkness into the light, I beg you to answer "yes" when your infusion nurse, or anyone, asks that question. I beg you to talk to a friend, a co-worker, cancer buddy – seek out your Pastor, Imam, Rabbi, Reverend, Priest and give yourself to healing comfort. While you can understand the despair, you don't have to give in to it. Give it to God and let him carry you and your burden for a while. You'll walk on your own strength again, soon. I promise.

Is it Cancer, Is it Cancer, Is it Cancer, Is it Cancer

As doctor's kids, I think my sister and I lost the panic button on our health. Even when it is something big, I rarely have sought out medical care. Having inherited my Dad's spinal disc issues, I have one in my neck, one in the middle of my back and one above my hip, all right side, that have given me issues for 25 years. Only when I was in law school and not able to stand upright when working through the practicum for Trial Advocacy did I seek medical treatment – steroid for inflammation and muscle relaxers to allow the disc to ease itself into my tight back.

During my third year in Law School, I suddenly lost vision in my left eye, followed by a warm sensation in my face. I'd had an awful headache for a week or so, but attributed it to stress, three jobs in Law School and reading too much. After I lost vision I thought "crap, I've torn my retina." Playing volleyball all summer, I naturally thought it to be an injury. Two weeks later, I finally went to the emergency room. "Hmmmm," said the attending, after looking in my eye, "may I bring a colleague?" I nodded. The next doctor said, "This is interesting. You know we are a teaching hospital . . . may I bring in a couple of my residents?"

"Aw crap," I thought, "this can't be good", but said "sure." I had a sizeable blood clot in the back of my eye. Either I'd had a TIA or Mitral Valve Prolapse or something else. An EKG later ruled out the valve, so the doctors settled on a TIA, with my birth control pills to blame. Although I still have a dead spot in my left eye, I simply went off of birth control and went on with my life.

The take-good-health-for-granted me died with my diagnosis. It never occurred to me that if took care of yourself, do your yearly mammograms, your yearly doctor's visits, twice a year dentists visits, colonoscopy at age 40, etc., that you could have a major health issue. I mean, it *did* occur to me that these things happened, but I always assumed good health for me.

It's a fine line to walk between being vigilant and being that crazy, hypochondriac patient that every doctor dreads and their front office dreads calling. Once in the ER with Bill for a gall bladder attack, I overheard the nurse comment on a patient in the next curtain over . . . "In here for the fourth time this week. Says it's his stomach this time. On Saturday he thought he had kidney stones." I don't want to be the patient who cries "wolf" so that when I have an issue, no one takes it seriously. But I also don't want to not raise an issue when I should – keeping it to myself and going down the rabbit-hole of worry is hard on the psyche. Karen Angel has been a good sounding board for weird things. I try not to bother her, but she gets serious when I neglect a detail – and not only because she documents like crazy for the National Cancer Institute. She really wants to know – and being a nurse, is dead on with assessments.

Once during my fourth round of chemotherapy, my body broke out in huge, welted rashes. Emanating from my elbows, my knees and around my stomach to my back, I could feel them coming on and then, there they'd be. For an hour or so, then they'd go away and come back a little later. Bill shot a picture of them and e-mailed to Karen. She immediately went through the "Did you eat something new? Did you wear clothes without washing them? Did you change fabric softeners? Did you change soap or shampoo?"

All answered to the negative. She called Dr. Lifeline's office and had them prescribe an antihistamine and then recommended topical Benadryl. It was gone in two days and never resurfaced again.

Immediately after I started to rebound from the therapies and was feeling stronger, I made an appointment with a great dermatologist for a skin check. I'd had a mole that was ugly and I had wanted removed for years. There is a three month wait to get into see the doctor. I agonized over that ugly mole for the entire wait, convinced it was growing, and that I'd screwed up and it was skin cancer. He cut it off on the spot, pronounced it ugly, but likely harmless and sent it off – Pathology confirmed it was just ugly.

Also, I'd been having problems swallowing in Spring of 2013. It felt like there was a pea in my throat, but food didn't get caught and it wasn't interfering with my breathing. Having had a friend with thyroid cancer 10 years before (she's doing great), I was convinced that that's what it was. I'd had my thyroid scanned before beginning the therapies and nodules in my thyroid were noted and likely benign. I thought that the radiation treatments had kicked it into overdrive and now I had thyroid cancer. Dr. Lifeline and Karen Angel had an appointment made with various imaging and a follow up with a well-respected endocrinologist. He laid the past thyroid scan film over the new one and agreed the nodules were likely benign and that there was no change in them since the year before. As an interesting aside, the awful acid stomach I had during chemotherapy has eroded the base of my esophagus a bit and the band of muscles (or something) inside, had been stretched from the inflammation. It's still there, but, if it's not fatal, I'll live with it.

Most recently, I went through a couple of weeks where I had a headache of and on for two weeks. Not constant through the day, but present at least some point during the day. Not raging, but present. I almost never get headaches . . . and I never wake up with one, but had a couple of days. Of course, I didn't want to verbalize my fears . . . Bill knew, just by reading my face when I mentioned it to him (too casually, probably). "My head hurts down into my teeth," I said. "It has for a week." He replied, "maybe you have a toothache that is hurting your head", knowing that I hadn't seen the dentist since pre-diagnosis. "I'm sure it's nothing."

When he left for work, I called our family dentist, Dr. Bud, who squeezed me in immediately. I told him my issue, he took multiple x-rays and couldn't find anything but normal erosion. No cavities, fillings in tact . . . nothing odd. He did point out a funky whitish line that runs along the top of the roots of my top jaw and noted that that was the bottom of my sinus cavity, and suggested that I might have a sinus issue. As I was leaving he said, "you never call to ask to be worked in, so I knew you were worried about something when you did." Bless Dr. Bud – he hadn't met "Hypochondria Beth" yet.

On my weekly check-in with Karen Angel, I gave her the Cliff Notes version, but didn't mention going to the dentist. She said that it may be Sinusitis, as the location of my headache was primarily under my eyebrows. She suggested an anti-histamine and an Aleve every 12 hours for a couple of days to see if that worked. Karen Angel offered to run it by my Yoda of an oncologist, Dr. Lifeline, but I don't want him to see the full gamut of crazy unless it's needed. And Karen Angel is usually spot on. Even though I didn't have a stuffy or runny nose, I started the regimen she suggested, awoke the next morning without a headache, started one mid-morning, took a dose of both again, noted the drainage down the back of my throat (and told her so) and was progressively better over the next few days.

Karen-Angel has become a dear friend. We know that, had we met outside of treatment, we would still be friends, as we have so much in common – Faith, family, philosophy . . . During one of our post-treatment lunches, she said that an older man who was a dear friend to her described life after cancer as sweet, but with a hard edge. He said that it was as if you're going through life and loving every minute, but with the image of an executioner's guillotine over your head, waiting to chop through the bliss. For me, that description is spot on.

I shared the latest with Deanna, who, ever herself, told me bluntly, with love, as I sat in my office before figuring out the likely culprit, "you need to stop. You can't do this to yourself. Unless you know it's something, you need to get on with it." I agreed, but said, "I know, but the thought of me botching my health again and leaving the Buddy is something I can't bear. I just can't. He won't reach his potential without me – whatever that is." She gave me that look, that those who know her recognize well and said, "you are fine and are going to be fine. You can't keep doing this to yourself."

I'm trying – trying to find that balance between crazy and alive.

Well, That's A Funny Name For It

The journey from chemotherapy to radiation and through the tunnel to the other side didn't go smoothly for me, of course. The big treatments were as smooth as can be, but getting to the drug therapy took some work. As part of the treatment protocol I was in, I needed to start the drug therapy within 12 weeks after my last round. When I went for the first month check-up after that round, and expected to get the prescription for Tamoxifen (as I was pre-menopausal), treatment threw me a curve.

Dr. Lifeline did his standard thorough check-up and then let me get dressed. When he came back in, he sat down and said, "I'm not going to give you Tamoxifen. With your history of blood clots, which is a potential side effect of that drug, I don't like the risk." I panicked. Tamoxifen was the talisman, the gold ring at the end of this ride. I know women who have been through *exactly* what I have who have been on it for nine years, 11 years, 13 years . . . . "That was 15 years ago. They thought it was birth control related." He asked, "did they test to confirm it?" The hospital hadn't. "I can't risk it for you," he said gently.

"What if I'm willing to risk it," I almost begged, the scream held barely below the surface. He said calmly that he wouldn't order it, but that we had other options. If I was in menopause, he could order Arimidex as drug therapy. Immediately I said, "How do we get me there?" From our discussion, I learned that there is a procedure called an Oophorectomy, where you can get your ovaries removed to trigger menopause in pretty short order. My task was to get the surgery scheduled (same-day surgery, through the belly button and two slits) sometime within the six weeks of eadiation, and come out with post-menopausal estrogen levels on the other side.

I swear, I wore out both the front offices of radiation and Dr. Glow. to get it going so I could come in menopausal during the 12 weeks' protocol for the clinical trial's time parameters of chemotherapy to beginning the drug regimen. Karen Angel, who hadn't made the one-month appointment, commented that you usually walk out with a prescription your first check-up, but assured me that the 12 weeks guideline was in place for a reason. She and Dr. Lifeline called the doctors leading my drug trial to make sure that an Oophorectomy wouldn't negate my continued participation in the trial (it didn't) and away I went.

The Oophorectomy was easy, compared to the rest of the onslaught my body had taken. The worst part was the sore belly-button (as I was warned). I had it done on a Friday and went back to work on Tuesday, working from home that Monday. And my reward at week 10 was post-menopausal numbers and my prescription of Arimidex. In fact, my estrogen levels were very low. Since this particular chemotherapy has a way of attacking estrogen, it had shut down my ovaries after the first round. I hadn't had a menstrual cycle since the previous September, so the Oophorectomy just finished the job. Also, since the chemotherapy had given me awful hot flashes and night sweats, Karen Angel opined that I had gone through menopause already. Having the Oophorectomy before my ovaries kicked back in saved me from going through it twice (Thank God). Another bonus, is that removing my ovaries eliminates ovarian cancer (of course) as some breast, ovarian and colon cancers are linked. Finally, it helps remove the fuel source for any cancer "floaters" that may be left behind. My cancer was estrogen fed – ovaries produce estrogen.

In the "be careful what you wish for" category, Arimidex is not without its issues. It is hard on your bones. I had a bone density scan before I started to start a base line, and will have it repeated periodically. On Karen Angel's advice, I take supplements to help ward off bone loss and try to walk more for weight-bearing exercise to strengthen my bones. No one in my family had osteoporosis, to my knowledge . . . but then, no one had had Breast Cancer either. My joints were initially so sore and swollen that it felt like what I imagine arthritis feels like. My size five and three-quarter wedding rink doesn't fit, so I've been wearing a size seven ring (tightly) on my wedding finger. My shoe size has gone from an eight and a half or nine to a 10. It's all good. The most irritating side-effect is the hot flashes. I'm already post-menopausal, how in the hell do I get the "sweat-running-down-my-face" hot flashes. At least once a day and out of nowhere. Nightsweats, too. My cancer-buddies on Tamoxifen say that they get them, too, so there's that.

Finally, Arimidex's potential side-effect of sleeplessness is full bore on me. I've always had insomnia – my Dad did, too. When I was in high school, I'd get up in the middle of the night and head down the hallway to watch some old movie until I was sleepy again. Invariably, Dad would already be there or would soon be. We watch whatever was on, he sitting on the coffee table, me lying on the floor beside his feet, with my head on the coffee table's bottom shelf. Since the mastectomy, I've not found a comfortable way to sleep. I was a "belly-sleeper" so that option is forever gone. I also can't shut off my brain from planning, worrying, praying, so the late night shows and I have gotten reacquainted. Adding

Arimidex ensures that I won't likely drop off to sleep the moment my head hits the pillow ever again.

    And with all that, I'll take it. I have a friend who can't wait to get off of it in the next year when her five is up. Me . . . I'm hopeful that I can elect to take it far beyond the safe zone. Whatever it is that can give me a hair's edge on survival . . . I'll take it. Remove another body part? Sure! Chemotherapy annually – leave the port in, I'm ready to go. As long as it keeps me here with my boys and alive to help David thrive, I'll do anything. Anything.

February 1, 2013

"I can't believe I'm going to get my first tattoos . . . at the age of 44." I thought. What a ridiculous thought. Still mind-numbed from the chemical cocktails I'd imbibed intravenously, I chalked it up to that. What is more likely, is that my personality, my absurd humor was trying to reclaim its foothold. Today I am going in to consult with the radiologist, to meet the treatment team, to see the equipment and, yes, to get tattooed.

I step into the radiation oncology office on the first floor of the same building where I have been treated for the past six months by Dr. Lifeline and have just completed chemotherapy. I've walked by the entrance to this last, active step in treatment so many times on this journey. Like a reward, getting to this step means that I've come through the worst of it and made it to the other side. Closing the door behind me, I survey the room. Much quieter than the Cancer Center and, although there are patients waiting for treatment, few of them have their support person with them. Almost everyone had a chemo comfort person, but few here. I'm even more relieved to be here, knowing that it's uniformly viewed as less arduous.

Once I fill out the paperwork and finally get back to Dr. Glow, I really try to focus on what he is saying. At every step of treatment, there is a new vocabulary, new equipment, a new process and new side effects. "There should be a 'cancer manual'," I think, trying to keep up.

"Radiation is not a requirement for treatment," Dr. Glow is saying, "nothing really is. As with any treatment protocol, there are *pros and cons for everything. Radiation is hard on the treatment site, but also hard on your body. The most arduous side-effect that most patients experience is fatigue, but there are others that we'll try to mitigate. The pro of radiation is that, for this treatment, it can cut the risk of recurrence in half, or down to around eight percent." That's all I needed to hear. I'm mindful that it's that low for the treatment area, and doesn't include reappearance elsewhere, but . . . if it drops it from 16% to 15%, I want it. I'll take every advantage I can get.*

Dr. Glow then looked at the site where the tumor used to be and the focus for radiation therapy . . . I'm so far beyond humility at this point that it doesn't even matter who sees. Soup-can expanders, scars, no nipples and all, being shirtless in front of new healthcare folks doesn't faze me a bit. His nurse has been waiting patiently throughout. What do I see in her? Her intelligent, light blue eyes betray nothing throughout, but . . . there is a "something else" in them. Dr. Glow finishes typing up the orders and answers my additional questions before I leave the consultation.

The pretty nurse takes me down the hall to get tattooed and measurements taken. She is around 60, petite, with short, almost white hair and so kind. We step into the "tattoo parlor" where two other women are waiting. Even as much as I've been through, every once in a while it feels like I'm a spectator in my own life, watching with great interest as a related, but distant, third-party. This is one of those times. The ladies strip off my gown again and, with gentle, but clinical, detachment, start going over what the machine is and does, the process, how the gel form is created, etc.. As the radiation penetrates beneath the skin layer into the chest cavity below, the Radiologist uses an inch or so thick, skin-like, gel overlay over the treatment area, called a "bolus" to concentrate the radiation to the area of concern and the tissues below, while (hopefully) protecting my lungs and other tissue below the site. "Bolus" is such a funny name for it – the word also means "chewed food", so the word-nerd side of me got a charge out of that.

One of the techs then explains that, once they slide me into the equipment in this room for measurements for the treatment site, they will tattoo three dots on my body as areas of reference for the radiation equipment later. Then, for each round, I will be lined up for treatment using those dots. At that moment, the pretty nurse, largely silent throughout the appointment, chimed in, "yours will look like this," as she pulled down the neck of her tunic and showed me a small, bluish marking in the center of her ribcage. And just like that, with her gesture of humanity and kindred solidarity, I felt an overwhelming peace and purpose. Side effects, choices for treatments, choices of treatment locations aside, I was <u>exactly</u> where I was supposed to be. Her treatment for breast cancer had been years before, and here she was, still living her life and helping others. That message had been the twinkle in her eye . . . the "I know what you're feeling and we'll take care of you." Irreplaceable, that understanding.

With that knowledge and under her watchful eye, the radiology techs slid me into the tubular machine. Reflected on the clear shield above, was an almost bull-eye grid of measurements, calculating to the nth based upon Dr. Glow's orders, where the radiation treatment should hit across my right chest and armpit. The tattooing itself was a non-even, due to the double-mastectomy which left me with little feeling and a pain-threshold much higher *than when I started. I assured these professionals time and again that it wasn't hurting and that I really couldn't feel anything.*

And I didn't – nothing aside from the belief that I was exactly where I needed to be for treatment and doing exactly what treatments that were right for me.

Radiation Therapy

Everyone I had spoken with prior to radiation therapy had opined that, after chemotherapy, radiation would be a piece of cake. Karen Angel even said that, for many of her patients, driving to radiation every day, parking, getting undressed, getting dressed, getting out of the parking lot, etc. was more of an annoyance than the therapy itself. She was right – they all were. Other than the grinding fatigue that compounded on the end and added to the chemotherapy fatigue, radiation therapy was a piece of cake.

I had been prescribed 30 doses, one per day (every morning at 7:30 for me so I could get to work on time), every weekday for six weeks. Starting in late January, 2013, until March 5, of that year, I had 25 sweeping treatments and a 5-treatment "boost" concentrating radiation on the spot where the cancer used to be. Every morning, I'd get undressed and into a paper top and wait to be called back.

Most mornings I had company waiting in the treatment anteroom beside the glowing photo of a waterfall. Some wearing the paper tops like I (men and women), some wearing paper pants, others with no hair or fuzzy hair from chemotherapy and some with slightly frizzy hair from radiation to their heads. All kind of folks coming from so many backgrounds, with different body builds, skin colors, ages, different kinds of cancers or other ailments at different stages and with different prognoses – we were all one, on common ground – we all wanted to live and would do anything for the brass ring of good health. Some of those with whom I waited wanted to talk, some didn't . . . I prayed with a few, wished "blessings" to them all and spent my time in the "sweep" remembering as many as I could by name, saying prayers for healing and giving praise that we lived in a country that had such life-saving, life-extending treatments. I didn't remember all of their names, but was comforted that God knew who I meant with each prayer, for He knows *every* name.

For each treatment, I would be led back to the therapy room, past a control room resembling that which you'd see on a movie about the moon landing. Not only did I check my name and treatment on the board every time, but this Radiation Oncology group also took my (wigged) photo during the tattoo session and had it on display at the entrance to the therapy room to match photo AND name. I would slide up on the table and get a pillow tucked under my leg for (relative) comfort and lift my right arm over my head, tucking another pillow there as well. The radiology technician would put the bolus over my right side – it was specially made for me from measurements. Using the tattoos, they'd line me up with the linear accelerator to make sure that I was getting treated in precisely the location prescribed by Dr. Glow.

My therapy typically took 15 – 20 minutes (I honestly don't remember precisely) and, although many describe the machine as a whir, to me, it sounded like (but didn't feel like) 1000 bees in a hive, changing course and regrouping again. I could watch the arc of treatment on the screen, gauging after the first few treatments how long until I was finished for the day. I used the time in prayer and contemplation, grateful for my life, grateful for treatments, grateful for my doctors and caregivers, for my Karen Angel, husband, family and friends. I'd pray for good days and quick healing for my fellow cancer survivors and warriors and for peace and comfort for all, no matter the outcome.

During the radiation treatments, I had the Oophorectomy, so, in addition to not being able to use my arms a lot to help climb up on the treatment table, for about a week post-Oopha, I couldn't use my stomach muscles either. Those poor folks . . . getting me onto the table, with legs and armpits I couldn't reach to shave, soup-cans under my skin, wig I had to keep tugging at, stiches in my abdomen, trying not to break wind with the effort (me, not them) . . . and not a word to dent what was left of my self-esteem.

Radiation is crazy-tough on your skin as it kills the healthy cells when it's killing potential demon-floaters. I was told to hydrate, hydrate, use moisturizing cleanser and to slather moisturizer as often as I could to the affected site. I chose "Aquafor" which is glorified petroleum jelly and slathered it liberally every morning after I left therapy, during the day if I needed to and more at night. Since it ruins clothes, I would keep strips of toilet paper stuck to it, then wrap an ace bandage to hold it in place. I smelled medicinal for weeks.

Every week or so, I had another nurse see me to check weight, side-effects and do a skin check. By the fourth week, I was definitely getting crispy, especially under my armpit. A friend of my Dad's wife sent two of the silkiest pillows to me. She had used them when she had gone through breast cancer 12 years prior. She had the same diagnosis, same stage and had the same course of treatments (please God) and, although she had only had a single mastectomy without reconstruction, she was doing great. Propping the pillow under my crispy armpit at night definitely helped me sleep, what little sleep I got.

Toward the end of my radiation cycles, right before I began the boost, I was talking to the nurse (who is just awesome). I was laughing that the chin hair was coming back more quickly than the hair on my head, but that my leg hair was much finer than before. She smiled and raised the leg of her scrubs to mid-thigh and pointed to a long, brown hair on an otherwise smooth leg. The nurse told me with a happy/sad smile that, after her bout with breast cancer nine years before, the only hair that grew back on her leg after chemotherapy was that one and she doesn't shave or pluck it as a reminder of her journey. The nurse had previously been an oncology nurse upstairs in the Cancer Center when, one day, as she held a patient's chart to her chest with her hands tucked under her armpits, she felt an enlarged node . . . and immediately knew what that meant. Although we had talked about anything and everything, we had never discussed it. Half laughing, half sobbing, I poured out my fear of the impending first three-month check-up after chemotherapy. "How do you get through wanting to check to make sure everything remains alright, but not wanting to find out if it's not?" I asked. She said that it would get better, but that it took years before she would even tell her husband that she was going for a check-up and didn't let him go when she did start letting him know. As much as I adore my husband, I got it. It's as if you love them so much that you want to spare them the first gut-punch and take it all, if you can . . . if it comes to that.

I left this appointment, again reassured. These amazing women are in my treatment world for a reason . . . they travelled down the same path that other women had before them, lighting the way for me and others, relighting the lamps that other women had lit for them, removing obstacles from my way to keep me moving ahead, safely on course. No matter what I am going through, my hopes and fears, there is someone to talk to who understands . . . personally, intimately, assuredly.

On my last day of radiation – day 30 – I got to my office to find balloons, banners, fliers and love. Although my work-family knows how private I am, they put so much effort into celebrating my last day of active treatments, bowling me over with kindness. Grateful, I accepted the good wishes and, only later, did I send out an e-mail of "thanks". Seemingly impersonal, I know, but they know me well enough to know . . . that I couldn't have spoken, couldn't have verbalized how much their love and support meant to me without cracking what fragile hold I retain on my emotions. Thanking them again here – for everything.

May 4, 2013

Today is my Bill's 58th birthday. It is also a rebirth, of sorts, for me. I had often attended the annual "Susan G Komen Race for the Cure" in Charleston in years past, although more in support of friends than an actual participant. This is my first year to attend as a Survivor – my first Race "after" . . . . I find it a wonderful blessing that my first "Komen" post-breast cancer falls on my sweet husband's birthday.

With a conflicted heart, both heavy and grateful, we decided to make this morning's events a family event. The Buddy will turn 10 on Tuesday, May 7th. Although he is minimally aware that I've been sick (with numerous appointments that he and Bill have picked me up from), he still doesn't know "cancer" and all the baggage that goes with it. As the Race is held at the State Capital, and the Buddy loves playing on the grounds, it didn't take much convincing for him to get up and go early on a Saturday. It also helped that the gym teacher at his school had pulled together a team of walkers who we helped sponsor. Bill was to run in the Race and our son and me experience the event and wait for his return.

It's a beautiful spring morning as we drive the three miles to the Capital. Even though we are early, we are forced to park two blocks away as other attendees are already streaming along the city's streets that run into the state complex. Setting foot on the grounds, there are tents everywhere and teams in brightly-colored shirts gathering for hugs and group pictures. Lining the Race route on Kanawha Boulevard are photos of tulips sponsored by folks as part of "Suzie's Garden" and in honor and in memory of those who have fought the fight. I recognize some of the names and am stunned. I've seen them in past years, but am now one of the survivors. The tulip sign that I sponsored doesn't have a name, but it does have a prayer – "From my tu-lips to God's ears." I'm crying so hard as I take a photo of it that I won't be able to tell until later if I've captured it.

My hair is coming in a little, so I have about an inch at this point. I've worn a black sweat suit and pink ballcap over the fuzz. Although I'm a little covered compared to most other folks, I'm still self-conscious about the soup cans and misshapen chest. I still haven't gotten used to them, even ten months later, and they feel alien. I feel alien, most of the time. Although there are many other patients I see during various appointments and treatments and with whom I e-mail, there is no one I see outside the clinical setting.

Winding our way to the front of the Capital, we arrive just as the loudspeaker announcement is calling for survivors to climb the steps for a group photo. "I can't," my mind screams, "I can't!" As usual, Bill senses my struggle and gently takes the Buddy's hand from mine, urging me toward the steps.

"Go on," he whispers, "you really need to do this – for all of us. Go take your place among the Survivors."

Tears streaming down my cheeks and with legs made out of lead, I head toward the steps for the group photo. All around me, moving in the same direction are so many others. Some with fuzzy hair, some with none and sporting scarves or hats, and some who are clearly veterans of the event. One woman has a tank top on revealing a scar on her back, likely from a latissimus dorsi flap procedure from breast reconstruction.

As I move with my sisters, my load lightens with each step and I am buoyed by the strength and purpose of our march. Still crying behind my sunglass, but no longer feeling alien, I take my place on the survivor's steps. One step below me, a beautiful woman turns in my direction and breaks into a welcoming grin. It's one of my nurses from radiology, the one who showed me her tattoo from the day when I received mine. Reaching up at me, she pulled me into a fierce hug and laughed, before turning back toward the camera as I sob with gratitude, both at her gesture and for God in delivering her to me when I needed her.

I see my guys in the distance near Boulevard. Bill is smiling in my direction, while the Buddy, seemingly oblivious, bops to the music playing. The fact that there are so many survivors is both thrilling and heartbreaking. It's sad that there are so many who have gone through the fear, anguish, pain and sickness that cancer – any cancer – can mean. It's also uplifting and inspiring that there are so many who have survived breast cancer.

Climbing down the steps, my journey back to my family is shorter than when I left them. I marvel at the celebratory atmosphere which nearly drowns out the fearful voices in my head. "Will I be one of the survivors next year? In two? In 10?" Meeting back up with my guys, we stand near the statue of Abraham Lincoln, the designated meeting place for his school Race team. One by one, the Buddy's teachers and parents materialize. Shyly, they hug me and fawn over my son, who (of course) thinks they are all there for him. One of the teachers is a cancer survivor and she gives me a gently smile, briefly squeezing my hand.

The team moves toward the starting line, ushered there by directions from the loudspeaker and the wave of other participants. Near the bright balloon arch is the WVU mascot, who has come to start the race with a shot fired from his musket. There are dance troops, a roller derby team, a hot air balloon and walls of pink as far as the eye can see. With the musket shot the WV "Race for the Cure" is off. Wave after wave of people pass the buddy and me, with the first group running and the slower movers settling into their paces. I spot Bill near the middle of the pack. He looks over at the Buddy and me and gives a wave. He is clearly crying as he moves down the road.

My son and I settle in along the river as we wait for Bill to complete the Race. Whereas in year's past I had participated, at this Race I fully understand. The "Race for the Cure" is held in earnest in cities, states and countries around the world. It isn't just a memorial for those who have lost their battles or an honor for those who have survived. It isn't even just a fundraiser for science and research in the form of a race to draw larger crowds. The "Susan G. Komen Race for the Cure" is more that all of that. These are folks on a personal mission to find a cure for breast cancer. If anyone is going to eradicate this evil, they will need to make it personal. It IS personal for all of us. The Race is personal for me in a way that it can't possibly be for someone if you haven't been through the fight. At that moment I am convinced that the Race will lead to a cure and I know that many who are here with us on this bright May morning are convinced of that, as well. It's why we're all here. I turn my face to the sky in gratitude for having the blessing to be here and a part of it all, while the Buddy plays happily near the flowers waiting for his daddy to return.

Reconstruction

Although I meant to document the date of reconstruction and beyond, that, too has hit a snag. So instead, this journey will be relayed in its milestones and setbacks – both ongoing.

During all the treatments, I had intermittent appointments with Dr. Bulldog to increase the size of the expanders. I was careful to schedule these during the upswing in both energy and immunity levels during chemotherapy, but, as fantastic as Dr. Bulldog and the nurses were during my appointments, it was still something else to think about and do during my fight for Survival. Dr. Bulldog had cautioned that radiation is hard on tissue and, about half the time, traditional reconstruction is difficult, if not impossible after treatment. I had three friends who were unable to have traditional reconstruction after radiation – one went ahead and had a tram flap procedure, borrowing fat, skin and muscle from her abdomen and transplanting it to her chest, and another said "screw it" and took out the implant when the irradiated side wouldn't heal. The third did a diep flap procedure, harvesting skin and fat, but no muscle, from her abdomen leaving her a beautiful, flat stomach as well as new breasts. She hates all of the scars. I've also had friends who had no problem – dice roll, I guess.

I was determined that I would be one of the lucky ones. I hydrated like crazy, wore bras that supported my new, perky implanted boobs, kept slathering the Aquafor . . . and kept hoping. The original surgery to switch out the expanders and put in the implants was mid-May, 2013. Compared to the double-mastectomy (and since I still had regenerating nerves), the surgery was nothing. I awoke with round, soft breasts instead of hard, egg-shaped soup cans and only small incisions on the sides. I slept more comfortably than I had in months and only took the pain medication for the first two days and then switched to ibuprofen.

Now we were cooking! The surgery was over well before our annual Kure Beach vacation, so I'd be healed in a bathing suit (with cup support) and in the water. It was a great summer. Suits fit better when you are a C-cup (even a fake one) than they do at DD, so I grabbed onto summer like an old friend and hit pools and the beach. Until Autumn.

I hadn't really had any issues until October 2013, when I noticed a half-dollar sized scaly patch on the "bad side", right around the boost site. As I would be on a conference call, I could poke that area and it seemed like the implant underneath had a bubble in the liquid. It just didn't feel right. I called Dr. Bulldog office and he got me in that first week of October.

"I don't like it," was his first reaction. "It looks like the skin there is really thin. I really worry if the skin breaks through, as the risk of infection isn't worth it." I sighed, resigning myself to another surgery either way, with the stubborn me wanting the months of expanders under my skin, fill-ups and annoyance to be worth it – and be rewarded with two boobs instead of a prosthesis on one side.

As if sensing my dejection, Dr. Bulldog agreed that we could try again. My other options were to scrap it altogether, try a flap procedure or take the implant out and give that side a break and try again later. Impatient me, I said, "When can we do it?" and so I had my second reconstruction on October 10. 2013.

I had my third six weeks later. The incision site never really healed from the second reconstruction, remaining a scab that grew wider and wider. On one of my three-month oncology follow ups, Karen Angel (never one to shy from a tough conversation) said, "You need to get that fixed. Even if it heals, it will be a tough scar." A week later, when I was getting out of the shower, I gently patted that area dry and the scab came away onto the towel. I called for Bill and had him look at the dime-sized hole it left. "What's that pink thing?" I asked. The implant was clear-ish, I thought. Calling Dr. Bulldog's office, he confirmed that I was seeing the implant, which becomes pink once exposed. So fewer than six weeks after the last surgery, I went in for number three.

For this surgery, I was determined to not fail. I had always plowed through things on shear determination. My body was going to fall in line, damn-it! Dr. Bulldog was resigned at this point and said "last time. If this doesn't work, there are other options, but we're not doing this again." I didn't want a flap procedure. My friend who had gotten the tram flap, despite having a fabulous set of new boobs and a tummy-tuck from skin and fat removal to transplant to her chest, said that it was still tough to sit up straight, as the transplanted muscle is one of those that helps you sit up. *Not* doing a tram flap.

The surgery was right before Thanksgiving week – perfect! I had that week off from work and we planned a trek to Canaan Valley for the mountains. Bill and the Buddy packed everything, loaded everything (including me) into the truck, and then unloaded me into the cabin at Land of Canaan. Dr. Bulldog had wrapped me tightly, had put in a smaller implant on that side (hey, we're all naturally lop-sided anyway) and we had put my right arm into a sling to reduce mobility. I slept with a pillow under that elbow to keep my arm from dropping and pulling on the skin and did NOTHING with my right arm until I returned to work. I was rewarded for all of this effort by keeping the implant . . . until March.

Dr. Bulldog had taken a new position a few states away with another plastic surgery group closer to his family and closer to his alma mater. The plastic surgery nurses were still at the multi-doctor practice (thank goodness), but I needed to see a new doctor from the practice. I had heard such great things about Dr. Phoenix (he was my friend Donna's surgeon and she loves him), that the choice was simple. I saw him for a follow up in mid-January, 2014, just to check on the surgery site and to get to know each other. I'm glad we did. I called his answering service on Saturday, March 22 - I could see the implant again and it was definitely infected. He immediately returned my call, called in antibiotics and saw me on Monday.

Defeated, I sat before him, tired and sore. Too dejected to even cry. "You know," he said gently, "the definition of 'insanity' is to do the same thing over and over and expect a different result. Let's give your body a break and we'll figure it out." And so, on March 26, 2014, I had my fourth reconstruction surgery in 10 months . . . well, technically, *de*-construction. I had been slated to give a presentation to clients with my boss on that day on a topic that I was largely responsible for. I had to call him the day before and tell him that he'd need to do the presentation without me.

I awoke after this surgery, deflated (literally, on one side), but somewhat relieved to not need to baby the right side any more. I had fought so hard to save the reconstructed breast that it giving up (for now) allowed me to shift my focus to more worthwhile battles. I was left with a wound on that side that would gradually heal over time, but I didn't need any (grenade) drains as there was little left to drain. I drained a small amount steadily for about three months, drained a little more in the morning when I awoke for another couple of months, then nothing at all. As I write, almost 9 months later, my half-dollar sized hole to my ribcage is about the size of a dime – it's slowly filling in from the bottom and sides.

During the early, post-surgery days, I would go through gauze a couple of times every day, trying to keep the area clean and dry. On one of my checkups with Dr. Phoenix, one of his brilliant, tenured nurses suggested, "We have some patients who use a sanitary napkin to catch drainage. Since it's absorbent and wicks moisture away, you won't need to change nearly so often." Epiphany! Down-side? My post-Oophorectomy, post-menopausal, Arimidex self *still* needs to buy feminine napkins . . . only now, I wear them on my chest. That tip has definitely helped in other ways as well. It gives me an extra inch of padding while the wound heals and, my skin is protected from frequent dressing changes. Having a latex-sensitivity issue means that I'm also sensitive to a lot of adhesives. I've found a cloth one at a local pharmacy (Fruth, for you local readers) that sticks well enough to leave for a couple of days, but not too much that it removes skin when I take it off.

One other scare, bears mentioning. On one of my post-surgery, six-month check-ups with Dr. Healer in August 2014, he took one look at the missing side with its wound and had an instant look of alarm. "Has Dr. Lifeline seen this?" he asked. I replied that he had, since I had had a three-month check up in late summer and was due for the next the next week. "What about Dr. Phoenix?" he asked. I again replied that I would go back every few weeks or so while I was draining, to check for infection and healing progress.

"I don't like it," he said. "I'm not doubting, but I'd feel better if we could biopsy around the site. Cancer cells inhibit normal cell growth and healing. I want to rule out anything sinister." I love his caution. I also thought that I'd be over the panic reflex by now, but there it was. Immediately the chant reared its head ("Is it cancer? Is it cancer? Is it cancer? Is it cancer?") We set the biopsy for his earliest available slot, while the schedulers did their magic to get me into the system. Of course, it was the following week, leaving the weekend to freak the hell OUT.

Going back in for the biopsy, it was the first time that I had been back to the Breast Center since that first biopsy two years before. Surreal. Filling out the paperwork, I glanced around the room at the others. Gauging by the looks on their faces, some were new to the terror, others apparently in for a yearly mammogram, and one (with a scarf over her bare head) sat in quiet contemplation, staring ahead. I wondered what they saw on my face . . . defiance that this will *not* be a recurrence . . . terror that it will be . . . resignation that this has become my new normal? I felt all of those.

Getting prepped and back in the biopsy room, I knew all too well how to lie, how to hold my arm and what was coming. The nurses and techs were kind and professional, but I still felt like I saw a twinge of pity when I removed my top to expose the quarter-sized hole that was there. Maybe it was just my imagination. Gentle Dr. Healer came in, promising that he'd biopsy under and around the open wound, so as to not disturb the edges of healing that Dr. Phoenix had worked so hard to achieve. He said that he was going to take substantial slices, though, to make sure he had good samples. Dr. Healer also said that he had a Radiologist standing by to analyze the first samples before I left, so we'd know one way or the other how to go. God Bless him for recognizing the terror of "the wait", but a part of me didn't want to walk out with the bad, if it was. The Faithful part of me was at peace. (Yes, I can be fearful and Faithful at the same time. The Faith is knowing that God has this no matter what. It doesn't keep me from fearing the "no matter what."). I had seen a double-rainbow in a magazine photo the night before my biopsy- a *double* rainbow over a thunderstorm showing two tornadoes. God's reinforcement to me.

Dr. Healer signaled that we were ready and started sterilization and prep. We bantered back and forth, tough teasing with a doctor who I've known for 16 years and who knows how to distract in a non-obvious way. Long needles numbing . . . I assured him that I felt very little, although I was getting some sensation back on that side.

"So," he said, "have I freaked you out, or are you all right?" he asked sincerely.

I held back the tears and the urge to scream "YES, YES, I'm freaked!", instead replying equally honestly that I appreciate his care and concern and that I knew he was doing the biopsy out of an abundance of caution.

Seven snips later and tissue onto prepared slides, he left the rest of his team to put me back together while he hand-carried a couple of the slides to the other doctor to read them. I was taken back to the first exam room while I waited an excruciating 30 minutes for Dr. Healer to return. When he did, I saw his cautious smile before I registered the rest of his face. "Now it's early," he started, "but there is nothing of concern." The radiologist said that he had seen extremely irradiated tissue, but no cancer cells detected. He noted that the radiologist was perplexed that he was standing over him and cautioned that there would be a second, more-thorough reading of the remainder of the slides, and that I'd hear by the end of the week. I told him that I'd wait for the follow up, but that I knew that I was fine. A few days later, I received the confirming call. All is well.

Please, God.

AFTERWARD

I don't like to leave loose ends, so there are a few that I need to tie up. I haven't seen angels since the time between my surgery and the first days of chemotherapy. I know they are there, but lending their light to those who really need to see and believe. I look, though, and smile at the memory. It sounds awful, but I hope to never see them again . . . at least not for a long time.

On August 2, 2013, my brilliant Dad lost his battle with cancer. We spent the final days at Hubbard Hospice House, he in peace and comfort and we in anguish. What a loving, compassionate, humane passing for him. It was tough to watch and, although I willed myself to stay with him and his loving wife in the final hours, it was hard to not picture myself there as well. I was there when he breathed his last and, as hard as it was, will forever be grateful to his wife for sharing that precious moment with me.

We had been warned that Dad's end was near, not only from the timeline that we had been given, but from my son's connection to him and to his Faith. Bill was going to take him home that evening, but David insisted on staying a little while longer. He left the kitchen/sitting area at Hospice where we had gathered for those last days and made Bill bring him into Dad's room. He wanted to hug and kiss his "Grandpa Doc" and tell him that he loved him. Dad passed fewer than two hours later. Bill later told me that, when David was trying to convince him to go into Dad's room, David kept looking out the large bay window. At one point, our 10 year-old, Aspie son looked into the sky and said, "Daddy, the angels aren't here yet for Grandpa Doc, but they are on their way. I really need to see him now." So Bill relented. I'm so glad that he did.

Finally, the rainbows. As I've said, they have always been my favorite Biblical sign. I know that I'm likely to notice them more now than ever for the portent that they bring, but I firmly believe that I am *given* them more than any other time in my life. I see them before *every* oncology follow up, before every test and before every procedure. *Every one.* On TV, in magazines, on the internet, in person …. never fails. I know that I will always see them, as I have throughout my life, and find in them the peace they bring for whatever may come. I DO hope that I don't see the angels again for a long, long time.